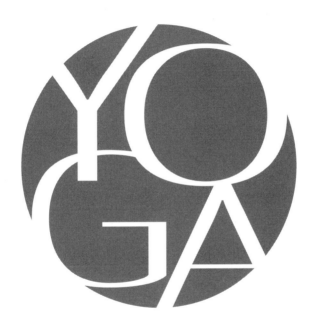

EXTREME
YOGA

**Challenging Poses
for a Cutting-Edge
Practice**

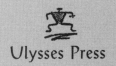

Ulysses Press

JESSIE CHAPMAN
PHOTOGRAPHS BY DHYAN

DEDICATED TO THE BALINESE PEOPLE
WHO SHOWED ME STRENGTH IS GENTLE AND SOFT.

Published by:
Ulysses Press
P.O. Box 3440
Berkeley CA 94703
www.ulyssespress.com

Library of Congress Control Number 2004101022
ISBN 1-56975-421-7

First published by HarperCollins Publishers, Sydney, Australia, in 2004.
This edition published by arrangement with HarperCollins Publishers Pty Ltd.

Printed in Canada by Transcontinental Printing

1 3 5 7 9 10 8 6 4 2

All photographs by Dhyan

Distributed in the United States by Publishers Group West
and in Canada by Raincoast Books

A Note from the Publishers:
Some of the postures contained in this publication should only be attempted under the
supervision of an experienced yoga practitioner. If in doubt, please contact your doctor or local
yoga center. If you have a pre-existing medical condition you should consult your local doctor
before beginning any course of exercise.

CONTENTS

NOTE FROM THE AUTHOR iv

1 INSIGHT INTO YOGA 1

2 YOGA FOR INNER STRENGTH, HEALTH & POTENTIAL 7

3 THE STRUCTURE OF YOUR PRACTICE 11

4 DEEP, FULL BREATHING 19

5 SITTING IN STILLNESS 23

6 WARM-UP SEQUENCES 33

7 THE POSTURES IN PRACTICE: 61
62 Arm-Balancing, 84 Sitting,
100 Lying-Down, 110 Backward-Bending,
125 Forward-Bending, 135 Inverted,
154 Partner

8 RELAXATION POSTURES 171

FINISHING PRAYER NAMASTE 177

ACKNOWLEDGMENTS 178

ABOUT THE AUTHOR & PHOTOGRAPHER 179

ABOUT THE YOGA MODELS 180

INDEX 182

NOTE FROM THE AUTHOR

There are times in our yoga practice when we need to hold back, to rest and restore the systems of the whole body, and there are times when we're overflowing with energy, yearning with our entire being to be more open, to learn more, to experience a deeper understanding and level of practice. This is when our practice becomes full or extreme. Our body and mind are in unison, and there is an equilibrium of softness and strength, flexibility and balance, will power and inner calm. We freely move into poses, or *asanas*, we never dreamed accessible to us, asanas we assumed would forever remain too challenging and advanced.

Extreme Yoga is best described as an integral practice, uniting breath, body, mind and intention. When we're in the "zone" or space of completeness, the very least of our concerns is performing the posture. Rather, we're one with the breath, and we're experiencing our body utterly. From this space, free of expectation and striving, we *yield* to the more challenging asanas rather than simply try to *do* them. We experience harmony — the very essence of yoga. The mind is not stilted by hardness; rather it is soft and open. The body is not dry with over-exertion; rather it is full with heat, yearning to expand and build. We experience the body's energies working synergistically, our natural ability to perform yoga asana improves ten-fold and we discover ourselves in postures we'd never dreamed of being comfortable in.

It is important to note that Extreme Yoga is born from a state of non-pushing, from a soft space where the body is open and fluid, and the mind empty of expectation. In this way, yoga teaches us that life can be lived best by doing less and being more. As our practice develops, our awareness of yoga and our self evolves and we discover the old adage that "less is more." We learn that by yielding rather than striving, we actually move further into yoga asanas than our mind could ever have anticipated. Yoga moves us beyond our own limitations.

The yoga postures, breathing techniques and meditations affect us in different ways and give us tools to use in our everyday life. When practicing yoga we are in a position to change. Learning to be in the postures requires certain levels of coordination, physical effort, mental focus and attention to breathing. These combined efforts stimulate personal development. In *Extreme Yoga* we're heightening our experience of the physical, mental, emotional and spiritual aspects of the self — and the unison of all its elements.

Physically we're challenged to stretch, strengthen, cleanse and tone from the inside out. We build a strong foundation of internal strength, from our inner organs and nerves out to our superficial muscles and skin. In Extreme Yoga, the body's systems are deeply stimulated and relaxed according to what is most needed, and the soft tissues and joints experience an invigorating massage. Our skin glows from continual cleansing of our organs and increased oxygen intake, and our eyes shine with good health.

As we become more flexible in our body with the practice of Extreme Yoga postures, we also become more flexible in our thinking and our mental approach to situations, making life more enjoyable. We experience increased mental clarity and focus. As we direct our awareness to the in and out breath in the postures, the mind is trained to maintain a single point of focus that becomes increasingly clear and sharp. We experience higher levels of concentration, and problems that once seemed overwhelming become more manageable.

Our emotional self is strengthened as well, and we find that we're less likely to be swayed by life's highs and lows. We experience an increased sense of inner peace, and relate to ourselves and others with more self-love. With the practice of yoga, and in particular the breathing and meditation practices, we develop a deeper connection within and cultivate a relationship with our true self. From this, self-awareness grows and we are more able to make choices in life that promote personal growth, happiness and potential.

Extreme Yoga details advanced postures for those who are yearning to go deeper. Most postures, however, can be modified to suit various levels of flexibility and strength. To begin your practice, establish deep, full breathing and then continue with some Warm-up Sequences from Chapter Six until heat is freely circulating throughout your whole body. Only practice postures that feel right for you on any given day and seek instruction from yoga teachers wherever possible to receive the gifts of their experienced insights. Use this book as an inspiration to deepen your understanding of yoga and the effects of the postures. Most importantly, approach your practice with a lightness and joy, avoid pushing or straining to get into postures and always modify the ones that are too advanced for your level of flexibility and strength.

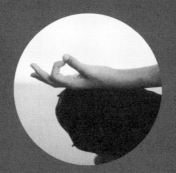

INSIGHT INTO YOGA

HE WHO KNOWS OTHERS IS WISE.
HE WHO KNOWS HIMSELF IS ENLIGHTENED.

Lao Tzu

THE YOGA JOURNEY

The yoga path is primarily concerned with developing a healthy mind and body, attaining self-awareness and fulfilling one's life potential. Its various practices and disciplines are available to everyone, no matter what their culture or the other paths they may follow.

The philosophy of yoga, which originated in ancient India, includes the practical disciplines of yoga *asana* (physical postures), *pranayama* (breathing techniques), *pratyahara* (withdrawal of the senses), *dharana* (concentration) and *dhyana* (meditation). The yoga journey also involves developing awareness on a universal and personal level through the *yamas* and *niyamas*, a series of ethics and disciplines intended to cultivate living in harmony with others and in oneness with our True Self.

Around 300BC, a yogi named Patanjali translated various Sanskrit texts and systemized yoga philosophy into the yoga sutras. These sutras, bite-size words of philosophical wisdom, were much easier to understand than the original texts had been, and made the yoga path available to a much wider Indian audience and, eventually, through the advent of travel and further translations, to people in other parts of the world too.

Practice Extreme Yoga by building on the foundation of your physical knowledge and on the understanding and integrating of yoga's philosophy. Do this and your core experience of yoga will shine through you. Remember that asana practice is a part of the whole system of yoga, and Extreme Yoga practiced without an awareness of this system becomes mere calisthenics. Be receptive to the wisdom of yoga, however, and you'll reflect the extreme richness of the practice on all levels of your life.

INTEGRATING YOGA PHILOSOPHY

Although yoga philosophy is thousands of years old and some aspects of the beliefs, disciplines and practices described in the ancient texts may seem outdated, it has been successfully adapted to fit with contemporary culture, and is easily integrated into modern daily life. Yoga is not a religion. It is non-sectarian and non-dogmatic. The primary teachings of yoga are an intelligent system focused on cultivating a healthy mind and body and an awareness of our oneness with all that is.

THE BASIC SYSTEM

The ancient Indian sage Patanjali systemized yoga philosophy into eight paths or limbs: *yama*, *niyama*, *asana*, *pranayama*, *pratyahara*, *dharana*, *dhyana*, *samadhi*. These limbs each express a different aspect of yoga and together make up the path or yoga practice that unfolds the physical, mental, emotional and spiritual levels of our being.

YAMA

These are ethical disciplines that relate to how we can live in a shared world with peace and integrity. There are five aspects.

AHIMSA —— **non-violence or non-killing.** Based on a perception that wars are borne from self-righteousness, *ahimsa* ultimately challenges us to live from an understanding of love, not from the fear and anger that leads to misunderstandings and violence on personal and world levels.

SATYA — **speaking and living from truth.** Knowing and honoring our truth allows us to live together with less confusion and more clarity and understanding. Being in the presence of someone who speaks and lives their truth is not necessarily always comfortable but is truly inspiring.

A S T E Y A — non-stealing. *Asteya* inspires gratitude and teaches that we can aspire to more whilst cultivating discernment and honesty towards ourselves and others. We can harbor a love for simplicity and learn respect and discipline.

B R A H M A C H A R Y A — chastity. This involves the cultivation of our sexual energy for direction and use in many areas of life rather than losing it through sexual acts. *Brahmacharya* is not necessarily celibacy but relates to the non-scattering of sexual energy. Through conscious direction of sexual energy, we can access an endless source of inner power and cultivate our health and potential.

A P A R I G R A H A — non-hoarding. This relates to living a simple life without undue excess. Over-consumption can lead to dissatisfaction; living with just what is needed allows us to appreciate the simple things in life and lessens our attachment to material objects.

N I Y A M A

These disciplines relate to the individual and focus on living a healthy, fulfilled and masterful life. There are five aspects.

S A U C H A — maintaining a clean body and healthy environment. This discipline of purity and cleanliness extends to the diet, living habits, home and social habits, as well as the development of clarity of mind, self-discipline and discernment.

S A N T O S A — inner contentment. To be contented is to be grateful for what is. Contentment reflects inner peace and an appreciation for life, for who we are and what we have. *Santosa* involves a sense of non-separation from self and inner harmony.

TAPAS — **the practice of conscious effort and regular discipline to develop inner strength, willpower and wisdom.** A simple example of this is maintaining a regular yoga practice which, when accomplished, strengthens our mental power and the union of the body with mind and spirit.

SVADHYAYA — **continued learning and development.** This keeps us growing and evolving. Study of the self and observing our reactions to others and events around us are also relevant. *Svadhyaya* promotes the observer within who helps us change and be free.

ISVARA PRANIDHANA — **devotion and connection with a higher power, universal soul or "God."** This practice or essence involves the development of humility and openness, and promotes inner peace and a wonderful state of innocence.

ASANA

The word *asana* means "to be," in the sense of being in a posture, such as the physical postures of yoga as demonstrated in this book as well as in the many other different styles of yoga in existence. The *asanas* were developed essentially for the maintenance of a healthy mind and body, with each posture affecting the body, mind and emotions in a unique way and working as a pathway to balance and well-being.

PRANAYAMA

In the practice of *pranayama*, we develop breathing techniques that increase oxygen intake and strengthen lung capacity while also increasing the absorption of *prana*, or life force. In its simplest form, *pranayama* involves deep, full breathing.

PRATYAHARA

This is the practice of withdrawing from the external world and involves all of the senses. As we close our eyes, shut out sounds and focus our awareness within, we develop the ability to journey inward to where the true self lies, and cultivate a connection that leads to inner peace and increased self-love.

DHARANA

Following on from *pratyahara*, *dharana* is the ability to be completely internally absorbed and focused. This practice of single-pointed concentration stills the mind and leads to a profound quietness within.

DHYANA

Following on from *dharana* is *dhyana*, or meditation — sitting where there is no focus, just stillness; no thoughts, only emptiness.

SAMADHI

In this state of absolute personal freedom there is union of the individual soul with the universal soul. It is the practice of living at one with all that is.

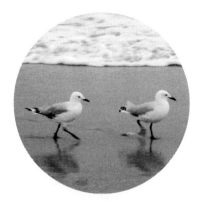

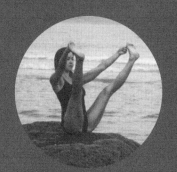

YOGA FOR INNER STRENGTH, HEALTH & POTENTIAL

LIVE AS IF YOU WERE TO DIE TOMORROW.
LEARN AS IF YOU WERE TO LIVE FOREVER.
MAHATMA GANDHI

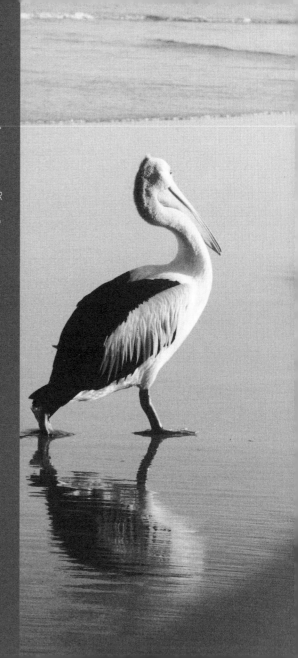

CULTIVATING INNER STRENGTH

WITH INTENSIFIED, REGULAR YOGA PRACTICE, AS WE MOVE FREELY BEYOND OUR MIND'S LIMITATIONS AND EXPLORE OUR FULLEST PHYSICAL POTENTIAL, WE EXPERIENCE INNER STRENGTH AT ALL LEVELS. THIS STRENGTH IS NO LONGER JUST A PHYSICAL ATTRIBUTE, TO BE ADMIRED OUTWARDLY, BUT RATHER RESTS IN THE KNOWING OF THE SELF. AS WE PROGRESS IN YOGA POSTURES, WE MOVE BEYOND THE PHYSICAL AND BECOME NOT ONLY COMFORTABLE WITH OUR BODY IN A WIDE VARIETY OF PHYSICAL POSES, BUT ALSO COMFORTABLE WITH OUR WHOLE SELF IN MANY AND VARIED LIFE CIRCUMSTANCES. WE EXPERIENCE CENTEREDNESS AND HAVE THE STRENGTH TO MOVE FREELY IN THE WORLD WITHOUT BEING THROWN OFF OUR PATH BY EVENTS OUTSIDE OF US. THROUGH OUR PRACTICE WE CULTIVATE AND MAINTAIN INNER STRENGTH AND ARE CONTINUALLY BATHED WITH A SENSE OF INNER PEACE.

YOGA FOR POTENTIAL

Yoga is a path of developing self-awareness and fullness of potential. In Extreme Yoga, as we journey more deeply into our practice, we move through different levels of opening and strengthening. When challenges arise, rather than giving up or straining to overcome them, see the challenge as the next step on your evolutionary path. If you learn to embrace the difficult phases with relaxed deep full breathing, you let go of pushing and straining and can rest softly in the initial awkwardness of the posture. With practice you will soon find that the posture that triggered the greatest difficulty will get easier and eventually may even become the posture you retreat to when needing a rest. When we take up the challenge of moving forward, rather than stagnating in what remains easy, we are saying yes to the many personal gifts of strength, awareness and understanding that yoga gives.

Inner awakenings are commonly experienced as we delve deeper into our practice, and these awakenings revive our strength to tackle new hurdles. Aspirations that had been put aside due to fear or a lack of confidence are reignited, and life becomes a synergy of development and discovery. With this integrated growth comes the potential to let go of negative habits and patterns that are no longer useful, and ultimately to make choices in life that serve our true passions and life purpose.

THE ROLE OF THE ASANAS

The intelligence of yoga is revealed in a simple and tangible way in the physical postures, or *asanas*. When we practice strengthening postures, our physical body systems naturally strengthen — the hormonal system is nourished, along with the nerves and soft tissues of the whole body; the immune system is boosted, increasing resistance to disease and the ability to heal; our bones are strengthened, preventing the onset of degenerative disease; and the brain is supplied with ample fresh blood.

Simultaneously, our mental state strengthens and our emotional being matures with the practice of the yoga *asanas*. People who practice yoga regularly will often comment that yoga helps them to be less attached to people and to outcomes, and to the emotions of happiness, sadness, anger or frustration. This reduction in neediness that happens in synergy with the strengthening of the physical self is one of the greatest gifts of yoga. And as peace within grows, this balanced way of being improves our quality of life and we can enjoy union with all that is with less attachment to outcomes.

The postures in this book were specifically designed with the interconnectedness of the whole being in mind, acknowledging the strengthening on all levels that unfolds with the development of physical strength. In the practice of back bends, for example, the chest, heart and lungs are opened, which consequently leads to more open and truthful communication and a closer relationship with our inner truth. In this way, yoga postures naturally strengthen the physical body from the inside out.

DEVELOPING AWARENESS IN EVERY MOMENT

Every part of the yoga experience is an opportunity to develop awareness — the movement in and out of the postures, for example. When moving beyond our mind's limitations into the zone of new postural experiences, we are effectively chipping away at layers and layers not only of physical hardness but also of hardened perceptions and beliefs. It's important to maintain a deep connection with the breath when working deeply so as not to "hit a wall" or cause injury through strain. In Extreme Yoga poses, remember to remain 100 percent connected to and aware of the body, the breath and the mind's attention working in unison to ride the wave of personal freedom.

When initiating movement, consciously engage your nervous system, which is where the body gets the orders to make movements. When you are working in a yoga posture, you are training your nervous system to activate and stimulate; in calming and relaxation postures and techniques, you are training your nervous system to relax at will. Having the ability to work with your body's energies allows you more freedom in life. If you can direct energy to where it is needed you will ultimately find the balance between the two energies of action and relaxation.

In the same way, we can work with the energy of the breath. Attaining a deep, full breathing rhythm is one of the most beneficial lessons of yoga. We can spend days or even months without food and even water but without the breath we would die almost instantly. *Pranayama* is the yogic art of breathing, or cultivating energy (*prana* — energy or life force; *ayama* — to develop or practice). Having breath awareness, staying focused on the breath in the postures, allows us to develop a deeper understanding on how "to be" in the postures (*asana* literally means "to be"), and in this way we learn when to activate and strive and when to just relax.

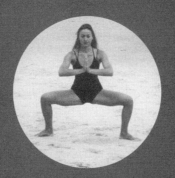

THE STRUCTURE
OF YOUR PRACTICE

**LET THE BEAUTY OF WHAT YOU
LOVE BE WHAT YOU DO.**
RUMI

3

THE ART OF VINYASA YOGA

VINYASA YOGA, OR DYNAMIC-FLOW YOGA, IS CHARACTERIZED BY THE MOVEMENT OR FLOW FROM POSTURE TO POSTURE USING A SERIES OF BREATH-BASED MOVEMENTS — A *VINYASA* (PAGES 14–15). CREATE YOUR OWN *VINYASA* YOGA CLASS BY COMBINING POSTURES IN THIS BOOK WITH A *VINYASA*. THE EMPHASIS IS ON MOVING THROUGH THE POSTURES IN A FLOWING WAY WITH THE AWARENESS ALWAYS ON THE "IN" AND "OUT" BREATH.

VINYASA YOGA WILL CREATE HEAT IN YOUR BODY, INCREASING YOUR CIRCULATION AND YOUR BODY'S CLEANSING PROCESSES AS WELL AS ITS FLEXIBILITY. YOU CAN ALSO ENHANCE THE DEVELOPMENT OF STRENGTH BY INCORPORATING A *VINYASA* IN YOUR PRACTICE. WITH REGULAR PRACTICE, YOUR BODY WILL NATURALLY REMEMBER THE FLOWING IN AND OUT AND THE MOVEMENTS BETWEEN EACH POSTURE WILL BECOME GRACEFUL AND LIGHT. THIS LIGHTNESS OF BEING WILL BRING A PEACEFUL EASE AND PRAYER-LIKE MOTION TO YOUR PRACTICE.

GETTING STARTED

Each posture in this book can be practiced individually or linked with other postures to make up a Dynamic Vinyasa class. Create a comprehensive practice by choosing a variety of postures from each section, including arm-balancing, sitting, twisting, supine, backward-bending, forward-bending, inverted and relaxation postures. Or create a theme for your practice, such as "Backward-Bending Postures." In this case, once you are sufficiently warmed up, you can move fluidly from a gentle backward bend to increasingly more intense forms of backward-bending postures. During the practice keep the heat flowing by incorporating the Vinyasa (see page 14).

WARMING UP

Before practicing the postures, begin by warming up with some *Surya Namaskars* (page 45). Doing five to 10 of these sequences quickly warms up the whole body and makes practicing the postures more comfortable. Starting with these sequences also helps to connect with deep, full breathing and develops strength throughout the whole body. If you require a less strenuous warm-up, choose another from the Warm-up sequences (page 33).

When you are sufficiently warmed up and feel centered, begin your practice with the chosen postures.

INCORPORATING THE VINYASA

To keep your body warm throughout your practice, include a *vinyasa* between some or all of the postures. In the sequence shown on facing page, the person is moving from *Trikonasana* to *Parsvakonasana* with a *vinyasa* in between.

1. Trikonasana
2. Caturanga Dandasana
3. Urdhva Mukha Svanasana
4. Adho Mukha Svanasana
5. Uttanasana
6. Masta Tadasana
7. Tadasana
8. Parsvakonasana

Make your practice ***vinyasa***-style by flowing through a sequence of postures to linking postures with the breath. A simple method to practice is: from the posture you are in, exhale to ***Caturanga Dandasana*** (staff pose), inhale to ***Urdhva Mukha Svanasana*** (upward-facing dog), exhale to ***Adho Mukha Svanasana*** (downward-facing dog) and then step or jump through to the next posture you will be holding for 5–10 breaths. Once you have finished the breaths, follow the above sequence again through to the next posture.

Putting a ***vinyasa*** between each posture with the breath creates a rhythmic flowing motion. Once in the posture, hold in it for about 5 breaths, or as instructed, and then move through the ***vinyasa*** with the "in" and "out" breaths to the next posture.

WINDING DOWN

Just as the beginning of our practice is focused on warming up, the ending is focused on winding down and relaxing. Always complete a practice with relaxation postures and ***Savasana*** (page 176), which allows your body to rest and you to reap the benefits of the whole practice. Without relaxation you could leave a practice feeling off-center and "wired." A deep learning experience and integration of the postures is gained when you allow sufficient time for warming up to begin a practice and relaxation to complete it.

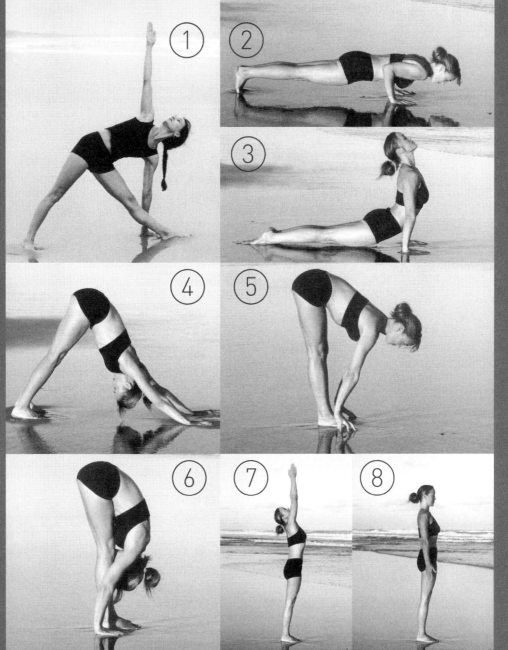

15

FINDING YOUR SELF IN YOGA
PRACTICE

It is best to practice first thing in the morning when the stomach is empty, the mind is peaceful and the external world is quiet. However, as we all have different schedules and lifestyles, any time put aside to connect with yourself in yoga is the right time, whether morning, day, afternoon or evening.

LIGHTNESS

Yoga is best practiced on an empty stomach. If this is not possible, allow at least two hours after eating before practice, so that your stomach is light.

COMFORT

Wear loose, comfortable clothing made of natural, non-synthetic fibers so that your skin can breathe through the fabric. Don't wear shoes or socks so that you have maximum contact with the ground. If possible, practice in a warm, dry environment out of direct sunlight and wind. A flat surface is good for balance and helps achieve correct alignment.

PROPS

Even, or perhaps especially, in challenging poses props assist us with balance, coordination, stretching forwards, opening the chest, inverting, twisting and more. Remember to have at hand any props, such as a strap, block or blanket, that help make your practice more fluid and comfortable. Even if you normally practice without the use of props, every now and again it helps to let the body be supported and assisted with props. A deeper level of opening often comes when we allow ourselves to ask for help or to be more comfortable in posture.

SACRED SPACE

To ensure a focused practice, find a quiet place away from any possible distractions. Take the phone off the hook, tell your family or housemates you're not to be disturbed, and be with your self totally.

BREATHING

Always breathe through your nose, unless it is blocked. Practice deep, full, slow inhalation and exhalation breaths. Aim to make the inhalation time equal to the exhalation time. Follow the breathing instructions given with the postures. Using the breath in practice will deepen your experience of the postures and will also help to prevent injuries. As a general rule, use the inhalation to lift and extend and the exhalation to soften and release downward.

THE POSTURES

The postures in this book aim to capture and reflect the essence of yoga at its fullest, suitable for advanced practitioners who have been practicing some time. For the postures you cannot do, look at them as offering you insight into yoga and find inspiration in the words and images. Only practice what feels right for you.

SAFETY

Be sensitive and listen to your body's needs. If you are menstruating, avoid inverted postures or those that are going to make you feel tired. If you are pregnant, consult a prenatal yoga teacher for postures specifically designed for the safety and comfort of you and your baby. While the practice of yoga is beneficial to health and well-being on many levels, if you have a known or suspected illness or disease, consult a medical professional before attempting the postures in the book, and see an experienced remedial yoga teacher for postures that will suit your individual needs.

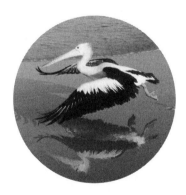

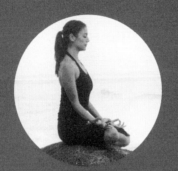

4

DEEP, FULL BREATHING

IMAGINATION IS MORE IMPORTANT THAN KNOWLEDGE.

ALBERT EINSTEIN

BECOMING AWARE
OF THE BREATH

The breath is the giver of life. As we inhale, we not only draw what the physical body needs, but we also take in an essence of life known as *prana*. This all-pervading life force, which is available to us at all times, is the subtle energy that feeds our soul. *Prana* gives us inspiration and connects us with our higher or true self. Obviously, therefore, we need to breathe well and deeply. When we move through our mind's limitations and are open to experiencing ourselves more fully in the following challenging postures, the breath becomes our most vital guide and protects us against injury and strain. Make time to develop a deep connection with your breathing before each practice and let the breath move you through it.

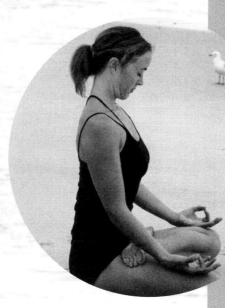

CULTIVATING DEEP, FULL BREATHING

SIT COMFORTABLY WITH YOUR BACK STRAIGHT, THE CROWN OF YOUR HEAD IN LINE WITH YOUR PELVIS. ROLL YOUR SHOULDERS DOWN AND BACK AND FEEL HOW THIS HELPS TO OPEN YOUR CHEST. REST THE BACK OF YOUR HANDS ON YOUR KNEES, YOUR PALMS FACING UP, AND TOUCH YOUR THUMB TO YOUR FOREFINGER; DOING THIS WILL TURN THE NERVE PATHWAYS GOING TO THE FINGERTIPS INWARD, WHICH HELPS TO INDUCE A CALM STATE.

21

As you inhale, focus on opening your chest, expanding the ribs out to your sides, and feel the intercostal muscles between your ribs expand. As you exhale, keep your sternum lifted and your chest open, and draw your navel back towards your spine, which will help to empty your lungs. Keeping your back straight and sitting erect, focus again on the inhalation. Feel your chest rising and expanding, and your lungs filling with air to the very top. Now slowly exhale, drawing your navel into your spine without collapsing your chest, and feel your lungs slowly emptying.

As you become more comfortable with this deep, full breathing, tuck your chin in slightly towards your neck, which will cause the muscles at the back of your throat to contract. This deepens the sound of the breath moving from the back of the throat and will feel as though you are actually breathing through your throat. Focus on cultivating this sound and begin to slow down the inhalation and exhalation breaths, which will increase your lung capacity.

Continue this conscious exercise for 5–10 full breath cycles or for 5–10 minutes if it feels comfortable. Focus on lengthening the inhalation and exhalation times, and on making them an equal duration. When you feel comfortable with deep, full breathing, use it while practicing your yoga postures. Breathing deeply and fully deepens your experience of the postures significantly and helps you to stay calm and relaxed.

If you need to, do the above breathing exercise lying down or leaning your back against a wall for support.

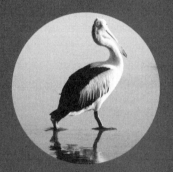

5

SITTING IN STILLNESS

I SHUT MY EYES IN ORDER TO SEE.
PAUL GAUGUIN

CONCENTRATION & MEDITATION

There are plenty of ways to experience what is known in yoga as *dhyana*, or meditation. You may have a passion that requires your utmost attention, such as painting, knitting or even dancing, and at times, after a long period of intense and focused concentration, your mind empties, you just go blank. This is meditation. The practice preceding meditation, that leads us into meditation, is known as *dharana* or concentration. You can practice concentration simply by sitting quietly and focusing on the in and out breaths. *Pratyahara* is also required to develop inner stillness; *pratyahara* is the withdrawal of the senses, the process of turning awareness inward, such as to simply close your eyes and shut out sounds and stop the sensation of touch.

The practice of *dharana* and *dhyana* often comes more easily when we are physically exhausted. Some people find a space of quiet and meditation comes naturally after an intensive work-out, such as a session of dynamic physical yoga postures. When moving deeply into Extreme Yoga postures, a sense of oneness and inner stillness is enhanced.

Practicing *pratyahara*, *dharana* and *dhyana* allow the mind a holiday from thinking. Afterwards, you feel refreshed, more energized and inspired. Do not be discouraged if at first your experience of stillness is not exactly peaceful; when we first begin to apply ourselves consciously to be still and develop a quiet mind, often the opposite happens and we are suddenly inundated with thoughts and plans. If this occurs, continue with your practice but don't set any big goals and approach your inward journey to stillness with joy and lightness.

SITTING POSITIONS
JNANA MUDRA
JNANA — KNOWLEDGE

IN THIS HAND POSITION THE FOREFINGER SYMBOLIZES THE INDIVIDUAL SELF OR SOUL WHILE THE THUMB REPRESENTS THE UNIVERSAL SELF OR SOUL. JOINING THE TWO PROMOTES THE INNER JOURNEY TOWARD TRUTH AND WISDOM.

POSITIONING: CHOOSE ONE OF THE SEATED POSTURES THAT FOLLOW. CLOSE YOUR EYES AND KEEP YOUR BACK STRAIGHT. BEND THE FOREFINGER OF EACH HAND AND PLACE IT BEHIND THE THUMBNAIL OF THE SAME HAND. STRAIGHTEN THE OTHER THREE FINGERS. THIS POSITIONING TURNS THE NERVE IMPULSES INWARD TO HELP DEEPEN RELAXATION.

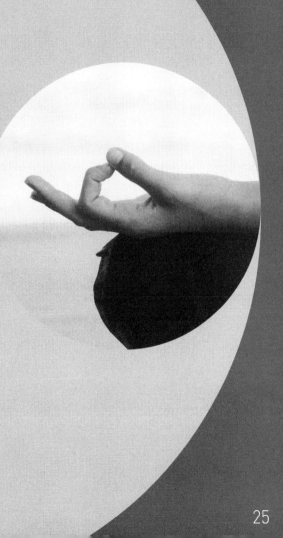

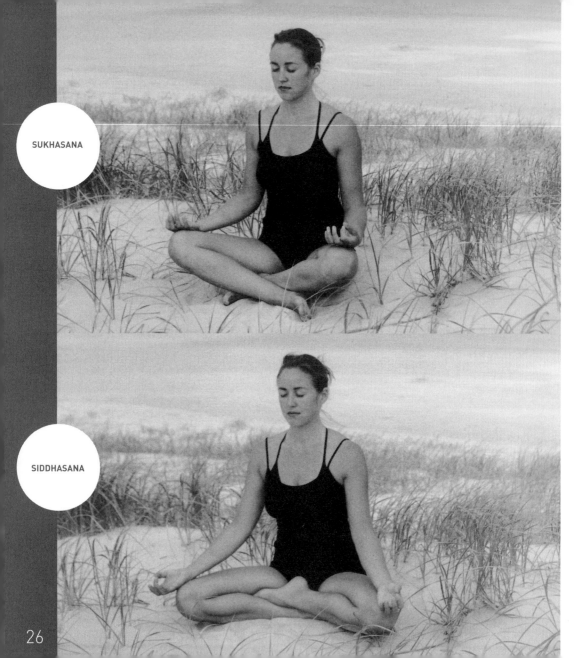

SUKHASANA

SIDDHASANA

26

SUKHASANA

SUKHA – HAPPY

POSITIONING: Sit in an easy cross-legged position with the back of your hands resting on your knees. Keep your spine straight and your head facing forward. Open your chest and soften your shoulders down and back.

VARIATIONS: Sit with your buttocks on some folded blankets for support. Sit with your back resting against a wall for support, keeping your spine erect. Wrap a cloth around your head to cover your eyes and help draw your attention inward. Wrap a cloth around your waist to help draw your lower back in and keep your spine straight.

SIDDHASANA

SIDDHA – SAGE
OR SEMI-DIVINE BEING

POSITIONING: Sitting with your legs outstretched in front, bend your right leg and place the heel of your foot into your left groin. Bend your left leg and sit the heel on top of your right heel, drawing it close into the pubic bone. Keep your spine, neck and head straight and in line. Rest the back of your hands on your knees.

VIRASANA
VIRA – A HERO
POSITIONING: Sit with your knees bent and your buttocks resting on your heels. Draw your knees and feet together and rest the backs of your hands on your thighs, relaxing your shoulders and arms. Keep your spine straight and your head upright.

VARIATIONS: If your ankles and feet feel tight, rest your legs and knees on a pile of folded blankets. Sit with your buttocks on a pile of blankets to ease any leg strain.

ARDHA PADMASANA
ARDHA – HALF; PADMA – LOTUS
POSITIONING: Sit with your legs outstretched. Bend one leg and place the foot comfortably into the groin. Bend your other leg and raise the foot up onto the thigh of your opposite leg. Release your upper knee toward the floor as you soften your hip. From this position, extend your upper body, lifting your chest, and straightening your spine and head.

NOTE: The half lotus position is a preparation *asana* for full *Padmasana* (page 30). The half lotus may be your limit for some time until your body loosens. Try alternating the leg positions to get opening in both hips.

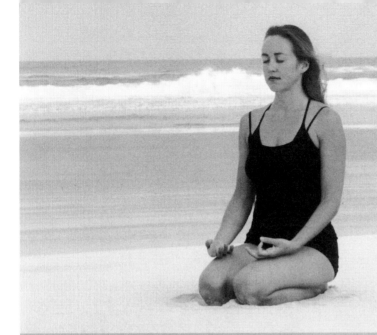

VIRASANA

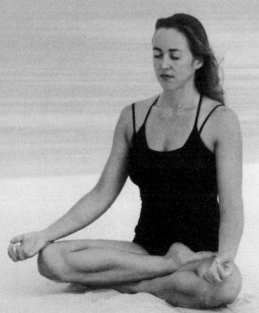

ARDHA
PADMASANA

29

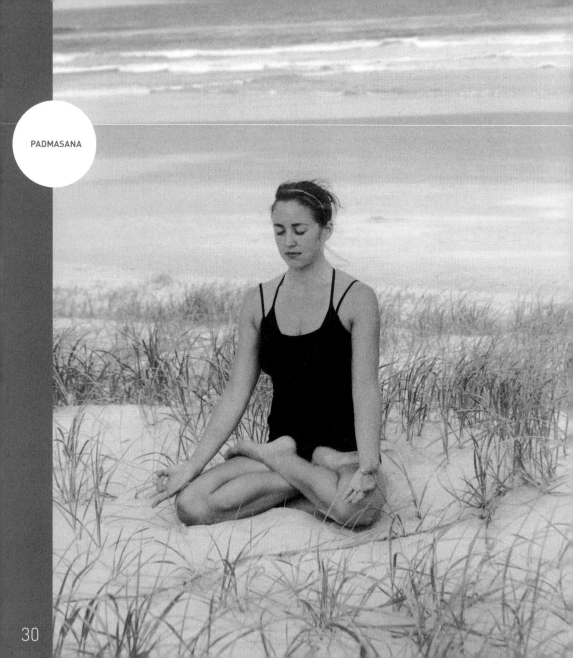

PADMASANA
PADMA - LOTUS

POSITIONING: Sit with your legs outstretched and your buttocks resting on a folded blanket. Bend your right leg and rest the foot on your left thigh with your right knee on the floor. Bend your left leg and place the foot on your right upper thigh. Draw both feet as close as possible into your body and rest your knees on or toward the floor. From this position, extend your upper body, lifting your chest, and straightening your spine and head.

NOTE: This position is ideal for sitting as it creates a stable base to rest in while the mind ascends to a higher realm of inner calm. However, it does require flexible hips and knees, so if they feel tight in this posture, use one of the other positions until you become more flexible.

INTEGRATING STILLNESS

Once you are in a comfortable seated position, begin to turn
your awareness inward. Close your eyes and consciously shut out any
sounds that are coming from around you. Reduce your awareness of your
entire external surroundings, including sensations such as the temperature of your
skin. This process of turning inward is called *pratyahara*, or withdrawal of the senses.

Now begin to quiet the mind's thoughts and chatter by choosing a single point to stay focused
on. Your single point of focus could be the awareness of the air moving in through your nostrils
and then out through your nostrils; without controlling the breath, just observe this movement of
air. Another common focusing method is to repeat the mantra AUM (pronounced "OM," this mantra
or sacred word symbolizes the origin of all sounds) in your head. Listen to your inner voice repeat
the mantra AUM over and over again. Repeating the same words overrides any thoughts or
distractions. Keep your inner voice loud and stay focused. This empties the mind of other thoughts.
This process of staying focused is *dharana*, or concentration. A steady, continuous flow of attention
on a single point is *dhyana*, or meditation.

At some point, and it may only last for a second or two, you drop into an empty space —
a place of nothingness that radiates from within and without, is universal and without
feelings of time or space. This is meditation. It can take much practice for you to
achieve *dhyana* — to empty your mind completely and be still. When you do,
you can begin to delve deeper and deeper into the quiet. This is the
journey into knowing your true self, where you are without
thoughts or ego.

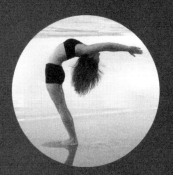

WARM-UP SEQUENCES

TO FIND YOURSELF BE YOURSELF.
SOCRATES

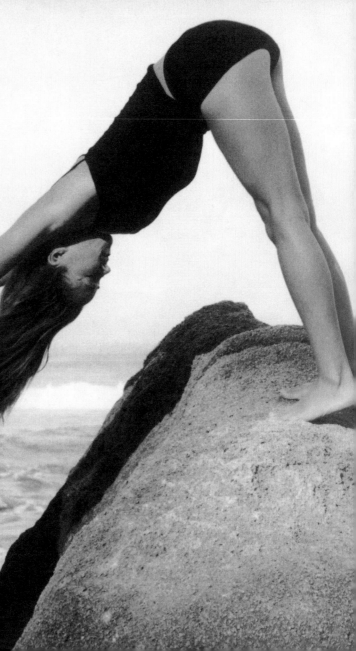

IN THE BEGINNING

THERE ARE A VARIETY OF
DYNAMIC STRETCHING AND
STRENGTHENING EXERCISES
THAT STRENGTHEN AND
STRETCH THE WHOLE BODY.
THE FOLLOWING SECTION
INCLUDES LIGHT WARM-UPS
TO CIRCULATE HEAT
THROUGH THE BODY, AND
MORE DYNAMIC SEQUENCES
FOR A MORE INTENSE
WARM-UP. WARMING UP
HELPS US TO CENTER WITH
THE BREATH BEFORE
ENTERING A DEEPER
PRACTICE, AND IS
ESPECIALLY IMPORTANT
WHEN APPROACHING THE
MORE CHALLENGING POSES
IN THIS BOOK.

In this section there are variations of the traditional *Surya Namaskars* (*surya* — sun or day; *namaskar* — salute or greeting). These flowing sequences stimulate heat throughout the whole body, increasing circulation and assisting with the natural cleansing processes. The *Namaskars* are ideal for morning practice, to awaken the whole body and mind, and also for general practice to increase flexibility and openness before moving into more intense yoga postures.

As we move with the breath, from one posture to the next, our whole being becomes a prayer in motion. When we know the full sequence and no longer need to think about what step to make next, we can turn the awareness inward and focus solely on the sound of the breath. As the body moves freely without thought, the mind empties and the practice becomes a moving meditation.

Start by familiarizing yourself with the sequences and the breathing rhythm. As a general rule, you inhale to lift and extend, and exhale to release and come down. Always breathe through your nose and focus on cultivating the sound of the breath moving from the back of your throat. In these practices, move in a flowing motion with the in and out breath from posture to posture, only resting longer in *Adho Mukha Svanasana* (the downward-facing dog *asana*). If you are short of time but are keen to practice some yoga before work, doing five to 10 *Surya Namaskars* with the breath will stretch and energize you for the day.

MARJARIASANA
MARJARI - CAT STRETCH

POSITION 1: Kneel with your hands shoulder-width apart and your knees hip-width apart. Inhale to lift your tail bone and arch your back as you look upward. Stretch your throat and lift your chest up through your shoulders. Gaze to your third-eye point.

POSITION 2: As you exhale, tuck your tail bone under, lower your head and lift your back up into the sky, stretching between your shoulder blades. Draw your navel back into your spine and gaze to your navel.

REPETITIONS: Continue inhaling to position 1 and exhaling to position 2 for 5–10 cycles to flex and extend your spine and to create heat in your body. Practice with breath awareness and try closing your eyes to deepen the experience.

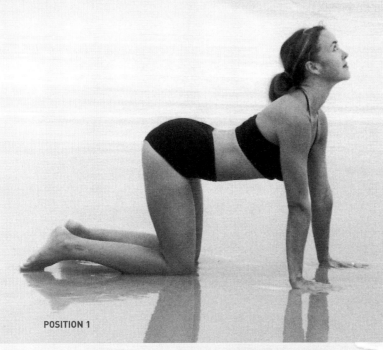

MARJARIASANA

POSITION 1

POSITION 2

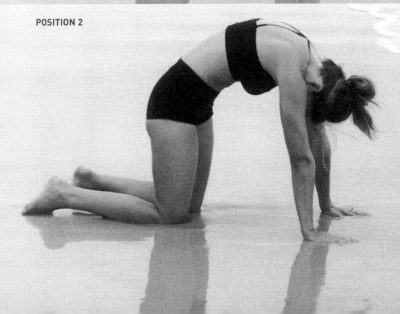

37

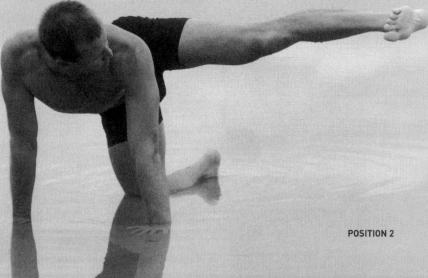

POSITION 1

POSITION 2

38

VYAGHRASANA
VYAGHRA – **TIGER**

POSITION 1: Kneel with your hands shoulder-width apart and your knees hip-width apart. Raise your right knee out to the side with the foot bent back toward the hip and the lower leg raised parallel to the floor. Hold for a few breaths.

POSITION 2: Inhale to extend your right leg out straight to the side, keeping the foot flexed and the leg parallel to the floor. Lock your knee and focus on a dynamic lift. Hold for 5 breaths and return to position 1. Release and change legs.

REPETITIONS: Repeat as many times as possible to tone the legs and buttocks and to create a deeply cleansing full-body warm-up.

CORE STRENGTHENING SEQUENCE

POSITION 1: Lie on your back with your legs pointing straight up, feet together. Inhale and raise your head and arms off the floor. Press your lower back to the floor and activate your abdominal muscles. Extend your arms out straight and keep your chin tucked in. Hold here for about 10 breaths (or longer if possible), strengthening the lower abdominal muscles.

POSITIONS 2 & 3: From here interlock your fingers behind your head and draw your right knee toward your left elbow, lifting your left shoulder blade off the floor as you twist to the right. Extend your left leg out and down about a foot off the floor and point your toes away. Hold here for a few breaths and then swap positions. Extend your right leg out straight and draw your left knee in, moving your right elbow toward your left knee and twisting to the left. Hold here for a few breaths and change positions again.

REPETITIONS: Move between positions 2 and 3 to strengthen and tone the lateral abdominal muscles.

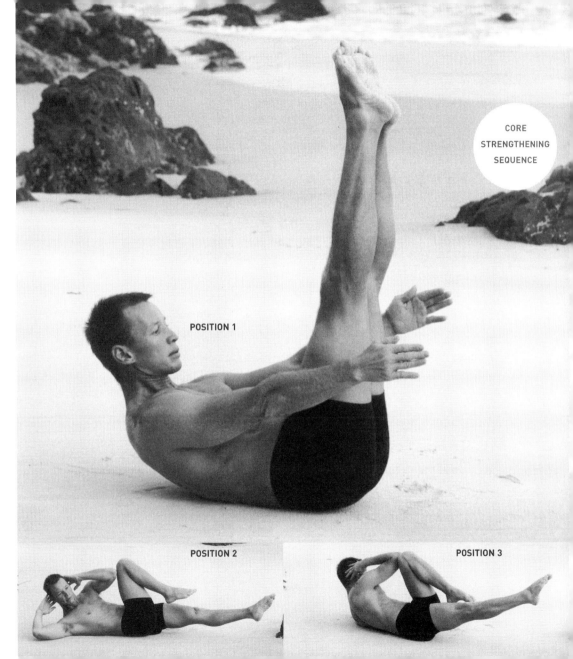

CORE
STRENGTHENING
SEQUENCE

POSITION 1

POSITION 2

POSITION 3

PARSVA HASTA TADASANA

PARSVA – SIDEWAYS; *HASTA* – HAND;
TADA – MOUNTAIN

POSITION 1: Stand with your feet together. Inhale to raise your arms over your head, bringing your palms together. Draw your navel into your spine and tuck your tail bone under slightly to support your lower back.

POSITION 2: Exhale to slide over to the right, stretching the left side of your torso. Stay looking forward and down, keeping your chin tucked in. Keep your arms extending strongly to the right behind the line of your ear and hips, parallel to the front. Keep your buttocks activated and your legs locked. Hold for 5 breaths. Inhale to release to the center and exhale to bend to the left.

REPETITIONS: Practice this side-stretching sequence for a few rounds to quickly heat up the whole body and develop a supple spine.

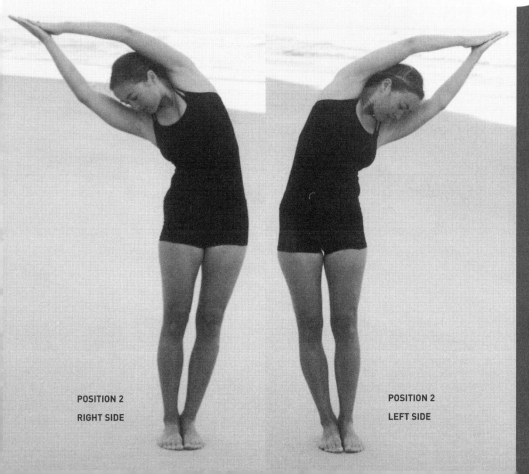

POSITION 2
RIGHT SIDE

POSITION 2
LEFT SIDE

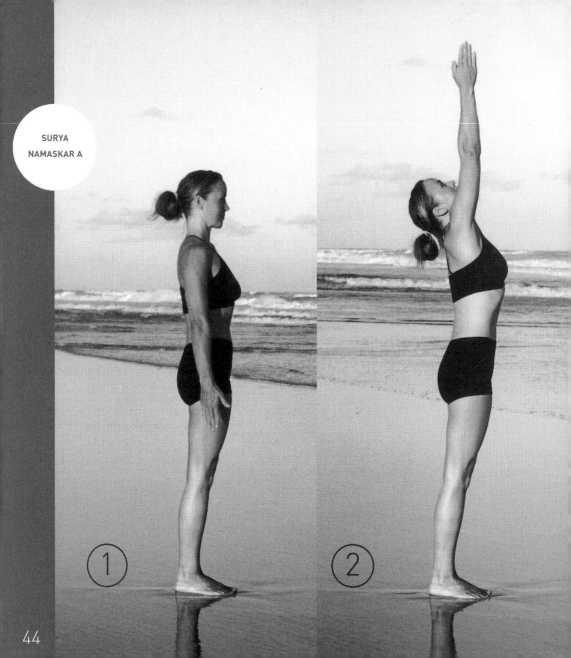

①

②

SURYA NAMASKAR A

SURYA – SUN; *NAMASKAR* – SALUTE

CENTERING: Stand with your feet together, the big toes and heels touching, and your body straight (if you are using a yoga mat, stand at the front). Bring your palms together in front of your heart. Turn your focus inward, developing concentration and inner quiet. You may like to chant AUM (pronounced "om") three times to begin your practice, or to simply focus on your heart center, radiating inner peace.

TADASANA 1: Release your arms down by your sides. Center your body weight evenly between your feet and the heel and ball of your right and left feet, spreading your toes wide. Lift your leg muscles; your kneecaps will lift as you lift and contract your thighs. Tuck your tail bone under slightly and lift up out of your lower back. Lengthen your whole spine upward. Roll your shoulder blades to the back and feel your chest open to the front and sides. Align the crown of your head with your pelvis. Bring your gaze to the tip of your nose. *Tadasana* means mountain pose — imitate a grounded mountain.

INHALE 2: Raise your arms upward over your head, bringing your palms together and looking at your thumbs. As you look up, lengthen the sides of your torso and push your heels into the floor. Keep your leg muscles activated and your spine lengthened.

EXHALE 3: Bring your arms out to the sides as you bend at your hips and drop forward and down into *Uttanasana* (*uttana* — extension). Bring your forehead toward your shins, tucking your chin in slightly and looking up toward your navel. If you have tight hamstrings or a sore lower back, keep your knees bent; otherwise, work your legs straight. Always lengthen your torso from the front rather than pulling out of the lower back.

INHALE 4: Look up, straightening your arms and bringing your gaze to your third eye (the point between your eyebrows). Lengthen the front of your torso and feel your spine elongate from your tail bone to the crown of your head.

EXHALE 5: Step or lightly jump your feet back into *Caturanga Dandasana* (*catur* — four; *anga* — limb; *danda* — stick). Keep your elbows in as you drop down into the pose. Squeeze your buttocks and draw your navel in to activate core strengthening. Your whole body should stay off the floor as you balance on your feet and hands; if this is not possible, rest your body down. Gaze to the tip of your nose.

INHALE 6: As you inhale, roll onto the top of your feet and lift your chest through your shoulders, balancing up on straight arms. This is *Urdhva Mukha Svanasana* (*urdhva* — up; *mukha* — face; *svana* — dog). If possible, keep your thighs off the ground; otherwise, rest them down. Lengthen your feet away, keeping your legs active, and roll your shoulders down and back, opening your chest. Focus on your heart opening here. Either face forward and gaze at the tip of your nose or drop your head back.

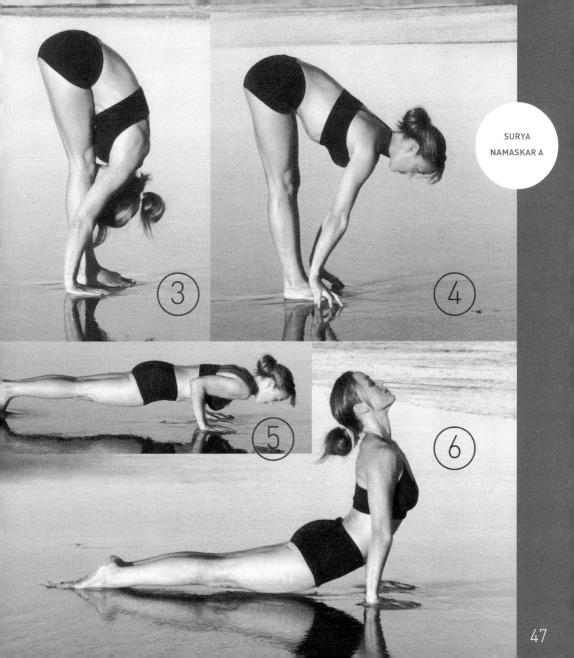

3

4

5

6

47

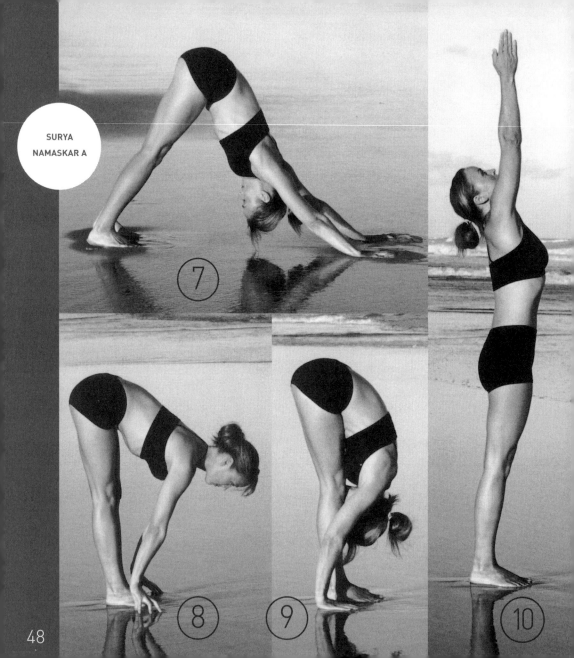

SURYA
NAMASKAR A

⑦

⑧

⑨

⑩

48

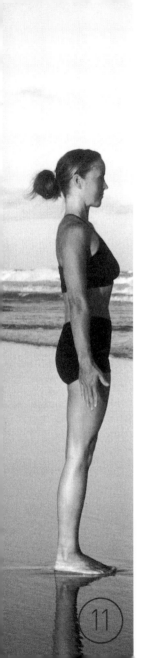

EXHALE 7: Roll over onto your toes and feet, lifting your buttocks and hips and lengthening up through your arms to *Adho Mukha Svanasana* (*adho* — downward; *mukha* — face; *svana* — dog). Focus on lengthening your arms and spine and the back of your legs. Bring your hips and buttocks upward as you drop your heels toward the floor. Tuck your chin in as you drop the crown of your head toward the floor. Your gaze rests between your feet on the ground or, if possible, toward your navel. Keep your gaze steady and focus on the breath for 5 breaths.

INHALE 8: Step or lightly jump your feet together to your hands and look forward (as in position 4).

EXHALE 9: Draw in your abdomen as you bend into *Uttanasana* (as in position 3).

INHALE 10: Extend your arms.out to the side as you lift back up to standing, bringing your palms together above your head and looking at your thumbs (as in position 2).

EXHALE 11: Release your arms down by your sides, coming back into *Tadasana* and bringing your gaze to the tip of your nose (as in position *Tadasana* 1).

REPETITIONS: Repeat the sequence for 5–10 full cycles with the in and out breaths to develop full-body flexibility and strength.

11

SURYA NAMASKAR B
SURYA – SUN; *NAMASKAR* – SALUTE

CENTERING: Stand with your feet together, the big toes and heels touching, and your body straight (if you are using a yoga mat, stand at the front). Bring your palms together in front of your heart. Turn your focus inward, developing concentration and inner quiet. You may like to chant AUM (pronounced "om") three times to begin your practice, or to simply focus on your heart center, radiating inner peace.

TADASANA **1:** Release your arms down by your sides. Center your body weight evenly between your feet and the heel and ball of your right and left feet, spreading your toes wide. Lift your leg muscles; your kneecaps will lift as you lift and contract your thighs. Tuck your tail bone under slightly and lift up out of your lower back. Lengthen your whole spine upward. Roll your shoulder blades to the back and feel your chest open to the front and sides. Align the crown of your head with your pelvis. Bring your gaze to the tip of your nose. *Tadasana* means mountain pose — imitate a grounded mountain.

INHALE 2: Raise your arms upward over your head, bringing your palms together and looking at your thumbs. As you look up, lengthen the sides of your torso and push your heels into the floor. Keep your leg muscles activated and your spine lengthened.

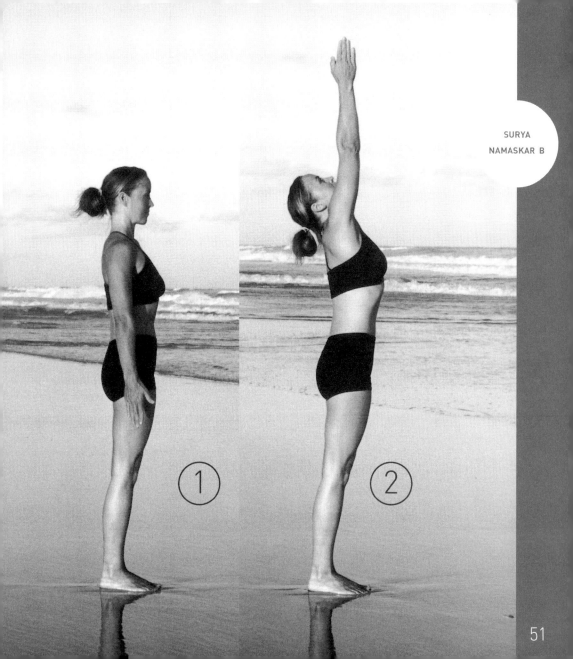

①

②

③

④

⑤

52

EXHALE 3: Bring your arms out to the sides as you bend at your hips and drop forward and down into *Uttanasana* (*uttana* — extension). Bring your forehead toward your shins, tucking your chin in slightly and looking up toward your navel. If you have tight hamstrings or a sore lower back, keep your knees bent; otherwise, work your legs straight. Always lengthen your torso from the front rather than pulling out of the lower back.

INHALE 4: Look up, straightening your arms and bringing your gaze to your third eye (the point between your eyebrows). Lengthen the front of your torso and feel your spine elongate from your tail bone to the crown of your head.

EXHALE 5: Step or lightly jump your feet back into *Caturanga Dandasana* (*catur* — four; *anga* — limb; *danda* — stick). Keep your elbows in as you drop down into the pose. Squeeze your buttocks and draw your navel in to activate core strengthening. Your whole body should stay off the floor as you balance on your feet and hands; if this is not possible, rest your body down. Gaze at the tip of your nose.

INHALE 6: As you inhale, roll onto the top of your feet and lift your chest through your shoulders, balancing up on straight arms. This is *Urdhva Mukha Svanasana* (*urdhva* — up; *mukha* — face; *svana* — dog). If possible, keep your thighs off the ground; otherwise, rest them down. Lengthen your feet away, keeping your legs active, and roll your shoulders down and back, opening your chest. Focus on your heart opening here. Either face forward and gaze at the tip of your nose or drop your head back.

EXHALE 7: Roll over onto your toes and feet, lifting your buttocks and hips and lengthening up through your arms to *Adho Mukha Svanasana* (*adho* — downward; *mukha* — face; *svana* — dog). Focus on lengthening your arms and spine and the back of your legs. Bring your hips and buttocks upward as you drop your heels toward the floor. Tuck your chin in as you drop the crown of your head toward the ground. Your gaze should rest between your feet on the floor or, if possible, toward your navel. Keep your gaze steady and focus on the breath for 5 breaths.

INHALE 8: Step your right foot forward between your hands so that your leg creates a 90° angle. Drop your left knee to the ground and position yourself over the back foot. Rotate your left hip forward so that your hips are parallel to the front. As you inhale, raise your arms up, bringing your palms together and looking up at your thumbs (or keep looking forward if this strains your neck).

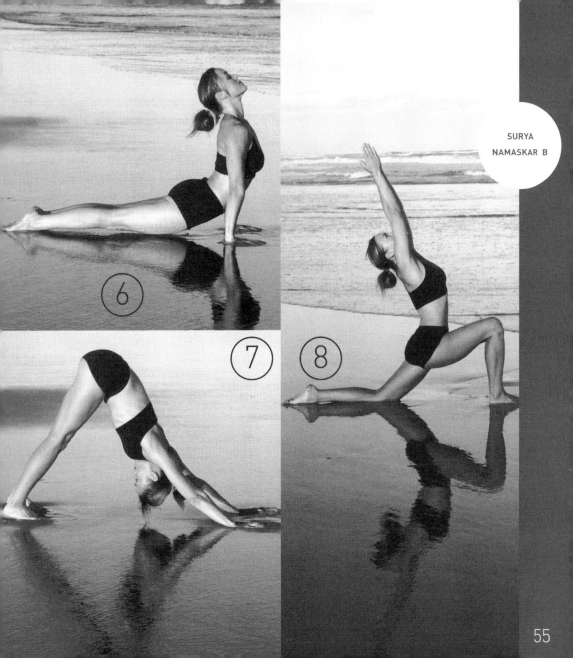

6

7

8

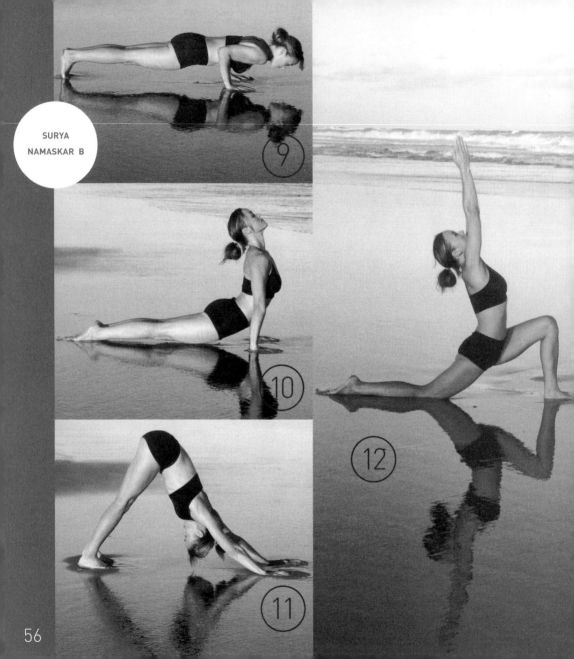

SURYA
NAMASKAR B

9

10

11

12

EXHALE 9: Place your palms on the floor beside your right foot, step your right leg back and, on the same exhalation, drop down into *Caturanga Dandasana* (as in position 5).

INHALE 10: Lift up into *Urdhva Mukha Svanasana* (as in position 6).

EXHALE 11: Move into *Adho Mukha Svanasana* (as in position 7).

INHALE 12: Step your left foot forward between your hands so that your leg creates a 90° angle. Drop your right knee to the floor and position yourself over the back foot. Rotate your right hip forward so that your hips are parallel to the front. As you inhale, raise your arms up, bringing your palms together and looking up at your thumbs (or keep looking forward if this strains your neck).

EXHALE 13: Turn the toes of your right foot under, step your left leg back and drop down into *Caturanga Dandasana* (as in position 5).

INHALE 14: Lift up into *Urdhva Mukha Svanasana* (as in position 10).

INHALE 15: Roll over into *Adho Mukha Svanasana* (as in position 11). Rest here for 5 long, full breaths. Focus on lengthening your arms and spine and the back of your legs. Bring your hips and buttocks upward as you drop your heels toward the ground. Tuck your chin in as you drop the crown of your head toward the ground. Your gaze should rest between your feet on the ground or, if possible, toward your navel. Keep your gaze steady and focus on the breath.

INHALE 16: Look forward and step or lightly jump your feet to your hands and look up (as in position 4).

EXHALE 17: Bend forward into *Uttanasana* (as in position 3).

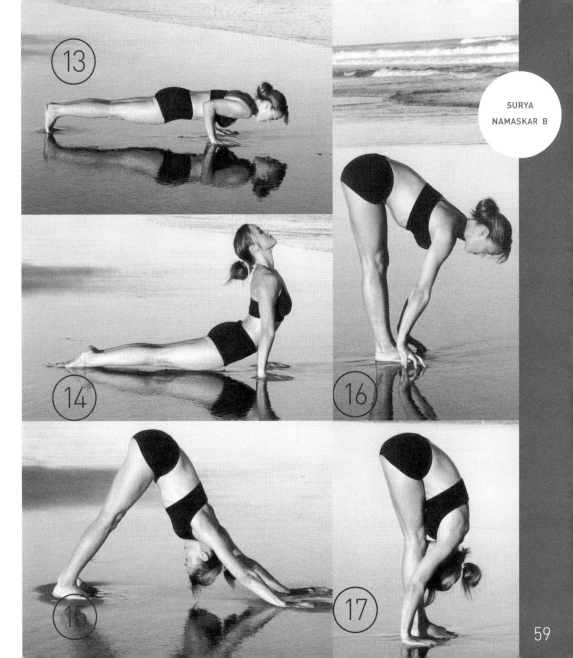

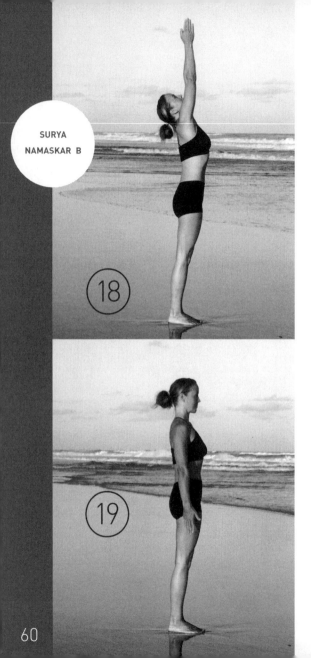

INHALE 18: To come up, extend your arms above your head and look up (as in position 2).

EXHALE 19: Release your arms down by your sides, moving into *Tadasana* (as in position 1).

REPETITIONS: Practice 5–10 cycles to warm up the whole body with the breath.

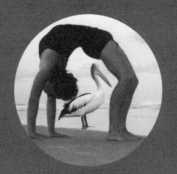

THE POSTURES
IN PRACTICE

THE OBJECT BLOCKING YOUR PATH IS YOUR PATH.
ANONYMOUS

ARM-BALANCING POSTURES

These dynamic arm-balancing postures not only help develop a strong upper body, they also invigorate your body, mind and spirit. Both external physical and internal emotional balance is required to be in these postures with calm and ease. Practiced regularly, these arm balances will not only strengthen your arms and tone your respiratory muscles but also increase your inner strength and self-control.

To practice these postures, center yourself with your breathing and get in touch with your abdominal muscles and core strength. Use the inhalation to lift up off the floor, hold the breath for a while, finding your balance, then slowly exhale and hold the balance for at least five more full breaths, breathing slowly in and out through the nose. Keep your arm muscles working evenly by spreading your body weight through the palms of your hands. Focus on keeping your gaze steady and directing your awareness inward to develop inner balance.

Although you will quickly build upper body strength if you practice these postures regularly, be careful initially not to topple head-first in some of the postures. If feeling unsure, place a pillow in front of you to soften the landing. Practicing on a sandy beach is another option. Avoid strenuous postures such as these if you are feeling tired or you have high blood pressure or heart problems. To keep straining to a minimum, focus on maintaining deep, full, slow breaths. As with all yoga postures, you will improve greatly with regular practice and focused intention.

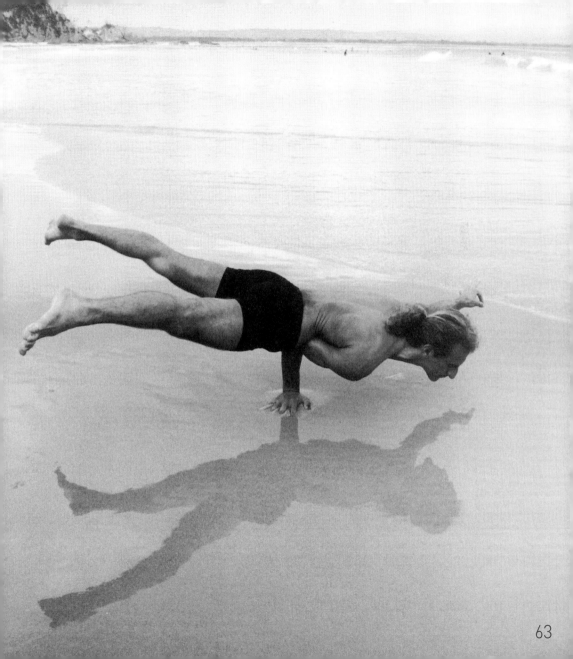

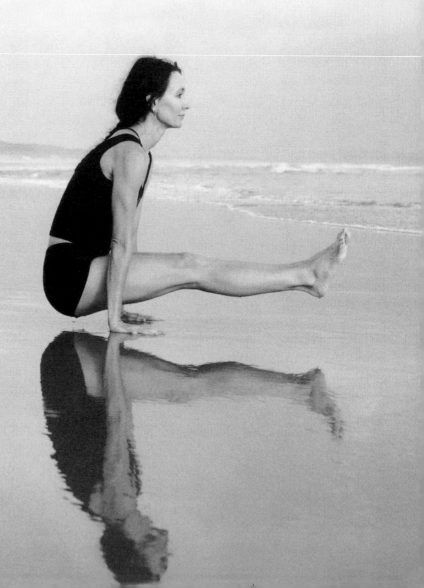

DANDASANA LIFT
DANDA – STAFF

Drawing from the vast storehouse of strength within you, lift yourself high and hover with the breath.

POSITIONING: Sit on the floor with your legs outstretched in front of you, your back straight and your chin tucked in slightly. Place your hands just in front of your hips on the floor. Lock your legs, activate your thighs and draw your kneecaps up. Activate your whole body and inhale to lift up off the floor so only your palms are in contact with it. Hover above the ground for as long as possible. For extra inner strength and lift, squeeze and lift your pelvic-floor muscles.

FOCUS: Activate your whole body and especially your arm and abdominal muscles to help lift and hold.

GAZE: Forward at eye level.

BREATHING: Soften your breath as you hover.

HOLD: Hover for as long as possible, then exhale to release down, rest and repeat twice more.

BENEFITS: Strengthens the muscles of the whole body and in particular the arms and trunk; develops core strength; strengthens willpower and mental focus.

BHUJAPIDASANA
BHUJA – ARM; *PIDA* – PRESSURE

Feel yourself growing from strength to strength as you strive to lift and hold with the support of your breath and arms.

POSITIONING: Stand upright, then bend your knees and place your hands directly behind your heels. Slide your upper arms as far as possible under your knees, so that your legs cross over your shoulders and your knees rest on your shoulders. Balancing on your hands, allow your feet to flop in front to the floor. Begin to shift your body weight back into the heels of your hands; as you do, the weight will naturally move from the feet and into the hands and arms. Allow your feet to naturally lift off the ground with this movement. Straighten your arms and press your palms firmly to the floor. Lightly cross your feet and look forward, dropping your buttocks down and lifting your feet higher.

FOCUS: Lifting your chest and straightening your arms.

GAZE: Softly ahead at eye level.

BREATHING: Long, slow breaths through your nose.

HOLD: 5–10 breaths then release, rest and repeat.

VARIATIONS: If unable to, do not cross your feet. Rest the heels of your hands onto the edge of a folded blanket to support your wrists if necessary.

BENEFITS: Strengthens your arms and wrists; develops a strong abdominal wall; develops willpower and mental calm.

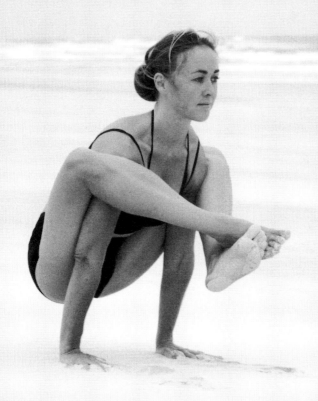

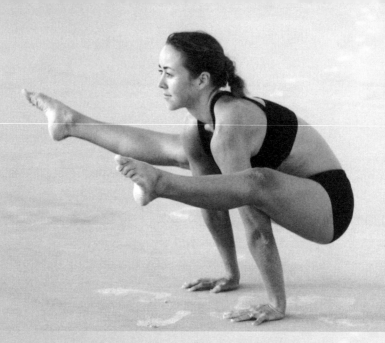

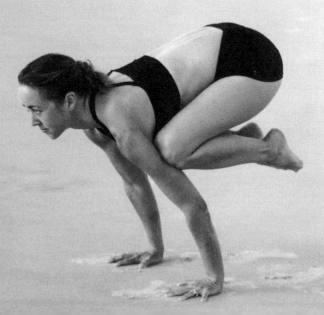

TITTIBHASANA — BAKASANA SEQUENCE
TITTIBHA – FLYING INSECT; *BAKA* – CRANE

To move from an extended flying position to a poised balancing posture requires strength, lightness and intention, and brings lightness and mobility.

POSITIONING: Move into *Bhujapidasana* (as shown on pages 66-67), then extend your legs out straight, keeping them off the floor and pointing your toes away. Keep your arms straight and your palms pressing firmly into the floor (as shown in top photo). Next swing your legs back and then bend your legs to press your knees into your upper arms as high as you can under your armpits (bottom photo). Move your body forward, shifting your body weight to find your balance. Press your palms down, straighten your arms and look ahead.

FOCUS: Developing a floating lightness as you hover supported by your arms.

GAZE: Softly ahead.

BREATHING: Soft, even breaths in the hovering position.

HOLD: 5–10 breaths then release, rest and repeat.

BENEFITS: Strengthens your arms and your whole torso, including the abdominal organs and nervous system; helps develop balance, willpower and focus.

ASTAVAKRASANA
ASTAVAKRA – INDIAN SAGE

The lesson in this challenging pose is that when you embrace your awkwardness you evolve through it.

POSITIONING: Stand upright, then squat down and place your right hand on the floor between your legs, your left hand beside your left foot. Wrap your right leg over your right arm, resting the back of your right thigh on your upper right arm. Lift your feet off the floor and cross your right foot over the left one, keeping them hovering in front of your right arm. When you have your balance, extend your legs sideways to the right, keeping the right leg crossed over the left. Lift up out of your lower back so your chest rises and begin to straighten your arms. Keep your legs raised and spread to the right.

FOCUS: Keeping your whole body lifted and your arm muscles working.

GAZE: Softly looking forward.

BREATHING: Soft, even breaths in the pose.

HOLD: 5 breaths, then release and change sides.

BENEFITS: Strengthens your arms, wrists and whole torso, especially the abdominal muscles and organs.

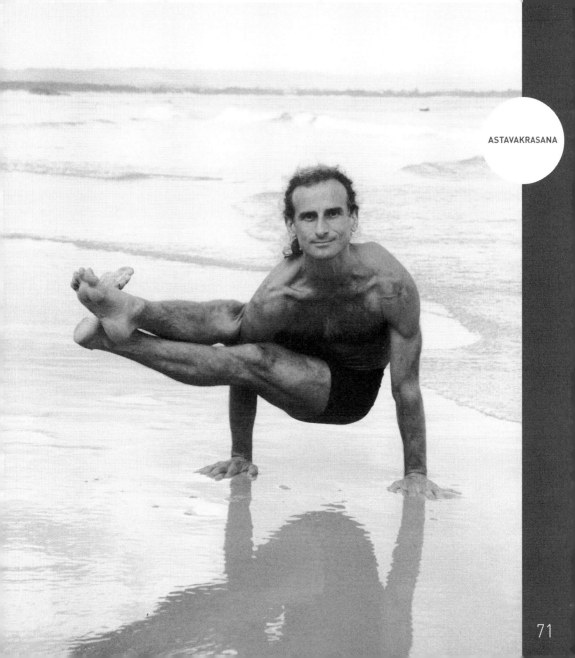

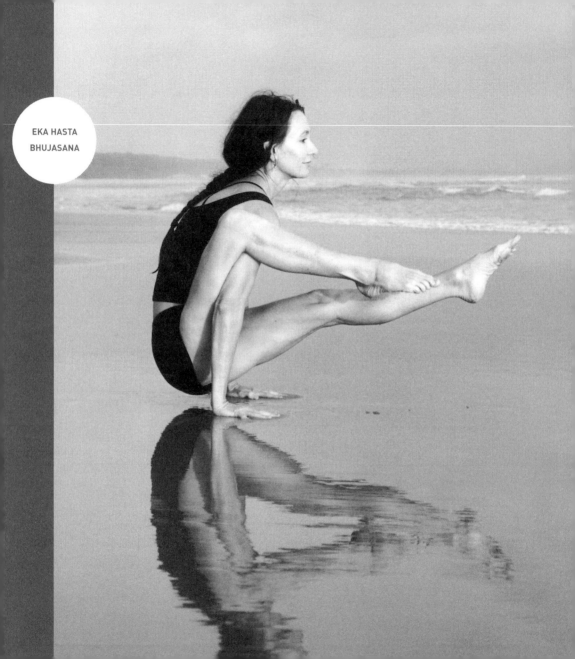

EKA HASTA BHUJASANA
EKA – ONE; *HASTA* – HAND;
BHUJA – ARM

Feel a strong sense of stillness in action as you point your toes away in this uplifting and energizing pose.

POSITIONING: Sit on the floor with your legs outstretched. Bend your right leg and press your palms to the floor beside your hips. Hook your right leg onto your right upper arm. Keeping your left leg extended and your arms straight, inhale to lift your whole body off the floor. Keep your right leg bent and pressed into your upper right arm for support and balance, and keep both feet pointing away. Squeeze and lift your pelvic-floor muscles to help keep your body lifted.

FOCUS: Keeping your arms locked and your palms flat on the floor.

GAZE: Softly forward.

BREATHING: Smooth, even breaths through your nose.

HOLD: 5 breaths, then release and change sides.

BENEFITS: Strengthens and tones your abdominal muscles and organs, arms, legs and your whole torso; helps develop willpower and endurance.

VASISTHASANA II
VASISTHASANA – INDIAN SAGE

This deeply toning balance challenges you to discover correct alignment, even weight distribution and inner calm.

POSITIONING: From *Adho Mukha Svanasana* (see position 7, page 54) roll over onto the outside edge of your right leg, resting your left foot on top of the right and balancing on your right arm (as shown in inset photo). Position your right shoulder directly above your right hand and lift your hips so that your body is in a straight diagonal line. Lift your left leg, catching the big toe of your left foot with the first two fingers of your left hand, and extend your leg upward, drawing your foot toward your head and continuing to lift your hips. Push out through the ball and heel of the raised leg and keep both arms locked. Turn your head to look up at your foot, tucking in your chin (main photo).

FOCUS: Maintaining a straight diagonal line with the bottom leg and torso; lifting up from the supporting hand; opening your chest.

GAZE: Up to and beyond the raised foot.

BREATHING: Softly and evenly.

HOLD: 5 breaths, then release to *Adho Mukha Svanasana* and change sides.

VARIATION: Look forward if you feel strain in the neck.

BENEFITS: Stretches your groin and inner leg muscles; strengthens and tones your whole spine, core center, legs and arms; helps develop inner balance.

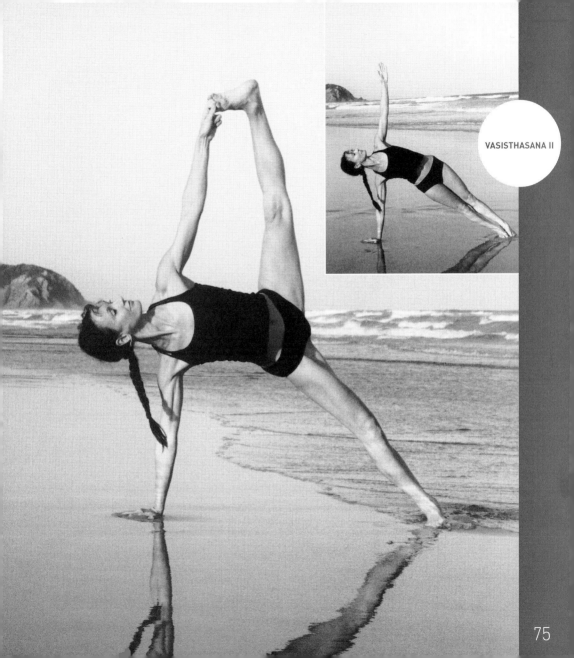

VASISTHASANA II

75

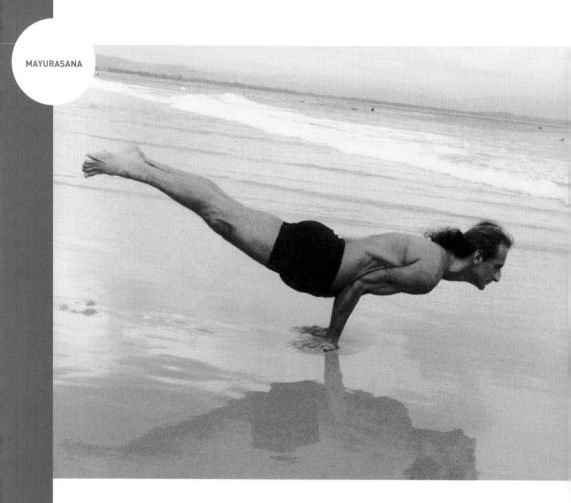

MAYURASANA
MAYURA – PEACOCK

Imitating the graciously light and composed peacock, in practice you will find inner balance, strength and a deeper self-knowledge.

POSITIONING: Kneel with your palms on the floor, your fingers turning inward to face your body, your wrists turned forward. Bring your elbows as close as possible together, then bend them in toward your belly, pressing your torso against your elbows and forearms. Straighten your legs behind you, with the tops of your feet on the floor. Lean into your bent arms and drop your head. When you find the strength, lift your head and feet so that you are balancing on your hands, your weight moving into your forearms. Keep your elbows in close against your torso.

FOCUS: Pointing your toes away from your body. Activating your whole body. Finding inner balance.

GAZE: Softly forward at eye level.

BREATHING: Focus on the soft sound of your breath as you hold.

HOLD: 5–10 breaths.

VARIATIONS: Strap your wrists together to keep your arms in close. Rest your raised feet against a wall behind you if necessary, until you build up enough strength to balance freely.

BENEFITS: Stimulates digestion and blood flow to the abdomen; strengthens the whole body, especially your arms and wrists; helps develop balance.

URDHVA KUKKUTASANA
URDHVA – UPWARD; *KUKKU* – COCK

As you develop inner balance and upper body strength you can move from posture to posture with pure intention.

POSITIONING: From *Salamba Sirsasana* II (as shown in inset photo), bring your legs in to full *Padmasana* by first bringing your right foot to the front of your left upper hip and then wrapping your left foot over your right foot to rest on the front of your right upper hip. Slide your feet closer together, then drop your folded legs and your head down. Place your head on the floor and rest your knees into your upper forearms. With your arms bent at right angles, lock your legs into position. Inhale deeply to lift your head off the floor and straighten your arms. Press your knees in toward your armpits, press your palms to the floor and lift up (main photo).

FOCUS: Straightening your arms.

GAZE: Softly forward.

BREATHING: Soft and even breaths.

HOLD: 5 breaths, then release and move back to *Salamba Sirsasana* II.

VARIATION: Alternate your left and right leg positions each time you practice.

BENEFITS: Strengthens your arms and upper torso; tones your legs; opens your hips; stimulates circulation to the pelvic region; helps develop inner strength, balance and coordination skills.

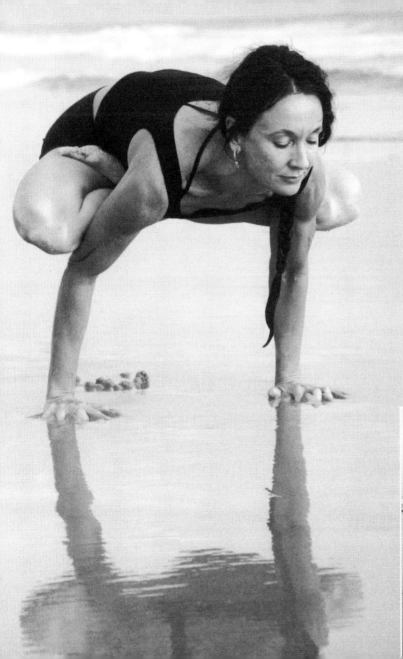

URDHVA
KUKKUTASANA

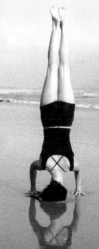

79

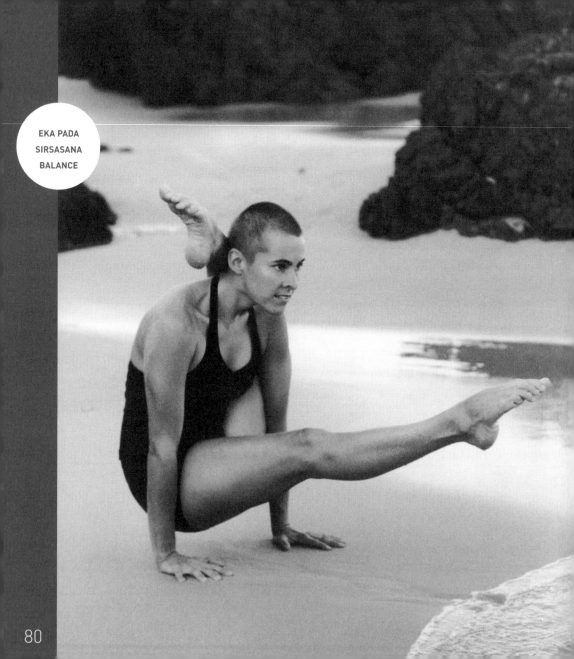

EKA PADA SIRSASANA BALANCE
EKA – ONE; *PADA* – FOOT/LEG; *SIRSA* – HEAD

Bathe in peace as you surrender to this pose, developing increased self-awareness, inner-strength and concentration.

POSITIONING: Sit on the floor with your legs outstretched in front. Raise your left leg, catching the ankle with your left hand. Extend the leg upright to stretch the hamstrings, then use both hands to bring the foot and upper leg behind your head to rest behind your neck. Roll your shoulders back and bring your left leg as far back as possible, your neck muscles working to slide the foot down and away from the back of your head. Lift out of your hips. Keep your right leg stretched forward with the toes pointed. Press your palms to the floor and inhale strongly to lift your body off the floor. Draw your shoulders back, creating space for your neck and head.

FOCUS: Keeping your arms strong; extending the pointed leg away.

GAZE: Softly forward at eye level.

BREATHING: Soft and smooth breaths.

HOLD: 5 breaths, then release your legs and change sides.

BENEFITS: Develops strength and balance; stretches your hamstrings; tones the leg nerves, spine and spinal nerves; strengthens your neck and head muscles.

DWI PADA SIRSASANA BALANCE
DWI – TWO; *PADA* – FOOT/LEG; *SIRSA* – HEAD

Entwining your body with your legs allows your spirit to surrender to the delicious experience of the unknown and unfamiliar.

POSITIONING: Sit on the floor with your legs outstretched in front. Raise your right leg, catching the ankle with your right hand. Extend the leg upright to stretch your hamstrings. Then use both hands to bring the foot and lower leg behind your head to rest behind your neck. When you have your balance, raise your left leg off the floor and use your right hand to bring your left foot behind your head to cross over the right foot. Use both hands to position your legs comfortably, then bring your feet further back behind your head, with your neck muscles working to slide your feet down and away from the back of your head. Place your palms on the floor beside your buttocks. When you are ready, inhale strongly to lift up off the floor. Keep your head as upright as possible.

FOCUS: Drawing your shoulders back to create space for your neck and head.

GAZE: Softly ahead at eye level.

BREATHING: Softly through your nose.

HOLD: 5–10 breaths, then release, swap leg positions and repeat.

VARIATION: Keep your buttocks on the floor if you cannot lift up.

BENEFITS: Stretches your hamstrings and inner legs; strengthens your arms, neck and spine muscles; helps develop willpower and mental focus.

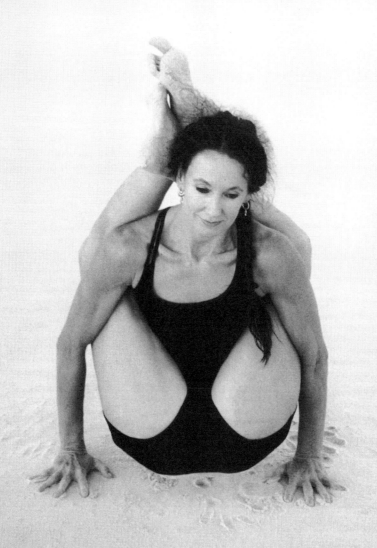

DWI PADA
SIRSASANA
BALANCE

SITTING POSTURES

Sitting postures enhance flexibility and inner calm. When sitting and focusing on the in and out breaths, you move deeper into the postures and learn to integrate your mind's intention with your body's flexibility and strength. Cultivating this mind-body connection is one of the sweetest qualities of yoga. As you abandon striving and pushing, you learn to expand your flexibility and strength through organic movements with the breath. Physically, the sitting postures work to open your hips, hamstrings, chest, shoulders and other tight areas in your body. They also enhance circulation to the pelvic and reproductive organs, increasing vitality and improving reproductive health.

Because sitting postures are inherently less dynamic than standing postures, they are more restful and allow you to turn your awareness and focus inward more easily.

Learn to work intelligently with your body in these postures and develop a supportive and nourishing practice. Utilize props whenever needed — wrap a strap around your feet to help hold your legs up, sit on blankets to help align your hips and use blocks for lift and support. You may also need to modify some of the postures to suit your flexibility and strength — keep your knees gently bent or only come halfway into a posture, for example. To make the practice more dynamic, move from posture to posture in the *vinyasa* style (pages 14–15).

Listen to your body and only do what feels right. Avoid strenuous sitting postures if you have heart problems, high blood pressure or nervous disorders. Be extra careful if you have knee problems. Check with an experienced yoga teacher if you are unsure of what is suitable for you to practice.

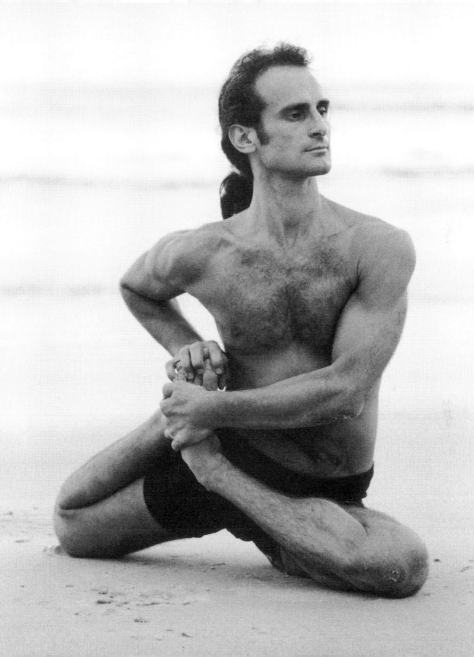

AKARNA DHANURASANA
KARNA – EAR; *DHANU* – BOW

Resembling the archer drawing his arrow back ready to strike, this dynamic *asana* promotes inner focus and graceful intention.

POSITIONING: Sit on the floor with your legs extended in front of you. Raise your right leg, bending your knee and catching the big toe with the first two fingers of your right hand. Lengthen out from the front of your torso and grasp the big toe of your left foot with the first two fingers of your left hand, keeping your left leg extended along the floor and activated. Keeping your chest open and lifted, begin to draw your right knee back, raising your right foot up to be beside your right ear. Inhale to lengthen upwards from the torso, exhale to draw your right foot back further, breathing into the inner leg stretch.

FOCUS: Opening the inner leg muscles of the lifted leg. Keeping your head upright and your chest open.

GAZE: Softly forward.

BREATHING: Smooth, even breaths.

HOLD: 5 breaths, then release and change sides.

BENEFITS: Flexes and stretches your leg muscles and hip joints; tones your abdominal muscles and organs; helps develop fluidity and ease of movement.

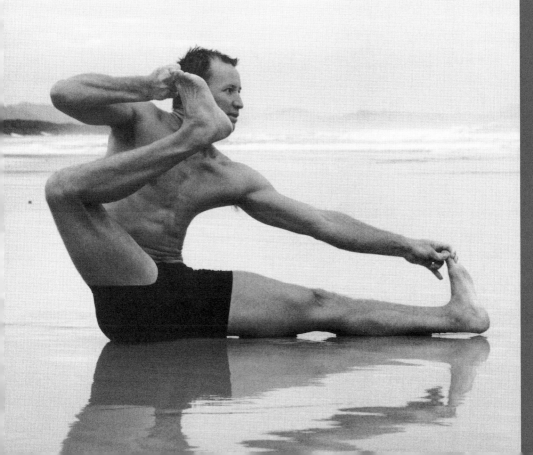

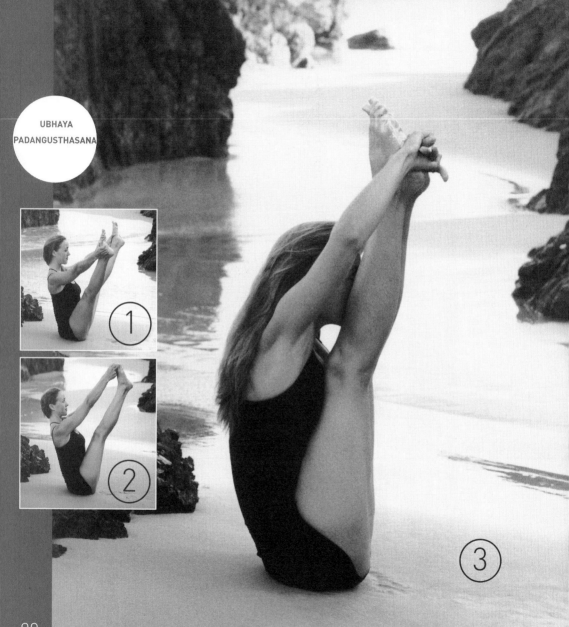

UBHAYA
PADANGUSTHASANA

①

②

③

UBHAYA PADANGUSTHASANA
UBHAYA – BOTH; *PADANGUSTHASANA* – BIG TOE

Move between these three *asanas* to inspire effortless balance and cultivate a yoga practice ripe with intention.

POSITIONING: Sit on the floor on your sitting bones. Extend your legs upward and hold the big toe of each foot with the first two fingers of the hand on that side. Lock your knees, drawing your thigh muscles up and in toward the bones to create sharply defined, compact, strong legs. Lift up out of your lower back and straighten and lengthen your arms to move your legs about 3 feet apart. Hold this first position for 5 breaths. Bring your feet together, lift up out of your lower back and balance in this second position, gazing forward, for 5 breaths. Draw your torso into your thighs, interlock your fingers around your feet and turn your palms outward. Point your toes away, lock your legs and keep lifting out of your lower back to hold this third position.

FOCUS: Lifting out of your lower back to keep your spine upright and prevent collapsing.

GAZE: Straight ahead or up to the toes and beyond.

BREATHING: Deep, full breaths.

HOLD: 5 breaths in each of the three positions.

BENEFITS: Strengthens your legs, knee joints, lower back and abdominal muscles; tones the nerves of your legs and spine; stimulates digestion; sharpens your mind and will.

KROUNCHASANA
KROUNCHA – HERON

Tastes of sweet, internal calm and deep quiet are yours in this beautiful posture that inspires fluid creativity.

POSITIONING: Kneel with your knees together and your buttocks raised. Turn your calf muscles out and tuck your tail bone under as you slowly rest your buttocks down between your heels on the floor, the top of your feet in contact with the floor. Inhale to unfold and release your right leg out in front. Raise that leg, holding the outside edge of the foot with your hands or interlock your fingers behind the foot with your palms turned out. Keeping your spine straight and your lower back drawn in draw your torso into your right thigh. Keep your right leg activated, the toes pointed and your back straight.

FOCUS: Lifting out of your hips; stretching the back of the raised leg.

GAZE: To the shin of the raised leg or beyond the pointed toes.

BREATHING: Inhale to lengthen from the front of your torso; exhale to draw the thigh and torso closer together.

HOLD: 5–10 breaths, then release and change sides.

VARIATIONS: Do not pull your leg into your torso if unable. Use a strap around your foot for support if necessary.

BENEFITS: Stretches the hamstrings and hips; strengthens the muscles of the front of the legs; tones the nerves of the legs; stimulates pelvic circulation; helps develop good posture and spinal strength.

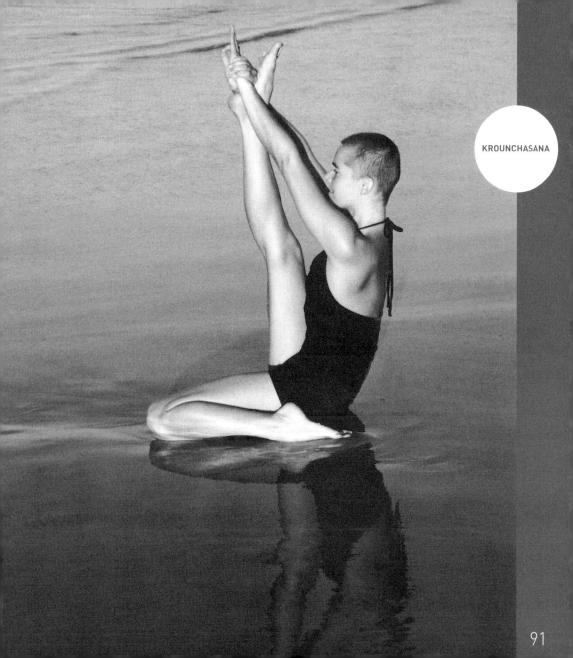

KROUNCHASANA

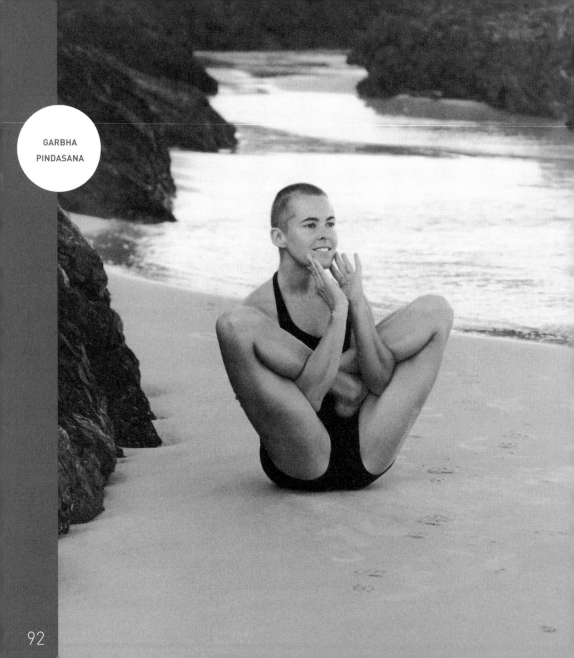

GARBHA
PINDASANA

GARBHA PINDASANA
GARBHA – WOMB; *PINDA* – EMBRYO

Resembling an embryo in a mother's womb, this pose weaves your limbs together to create a comforting embrace.

POSITIONING: Sit on the floor and raise your right leg, rolling your thigh outward as you place your right foot on top of your left upper thigh. Let your right knee sink to the floor. Raise your left leg and bring the foot to rest on top of your right upper thigh. Keep your spine lifting upward from your pelvic base. Slide your hands between your thighs and calves on each side (drip some water on your legs and arms before attempting the pose to make sliding your arms through easier). Lift your thighs off the floor so that you are balancing on your tail bone. Place your fingers on your chin, your palms facing upward. Keep your thighs close to your chest and your back upright.

FOCUS: Sliding your arms through your legs as far as possible; keeping your thighs close to your torso.

GAZE: Softly forward at eye level.

BREATHING: Soft and calm breaths.

HOLD: 5 breaths, then release and cross your legs the other way.

VARIATION: If you cannot slide both arms through, begin with just one.

BENEFITS: Nourishes the abdominal organs; opens your hips; stretches your arms and shoulders.

HANUMANASANA
HANUMAN – MONKEY

A powerful posture to invoke suppleness of the body, softness of the mind and lightness of the spirit.

POSITIONING: Kneel on the floor, your hands resting on the floor on either side of your legs. Step your right leg forward with the heel to the floor, the toes flexed back toward your hips and the back of your leg stretching away. Slide your left leg back, the top of your foot in contact with the floor. Lift your left knee and pelvis off the ground. Align your hips to be parallel at the front and lift out from your spine. Soften into the pose using the breath and begin to lower your groin closer to the floor, keeping both legs extending away from each other and your hips parallel. Keep your palms to the floor or, if you are comfortable, raise your arms and bring the palms together above your head.

FOCUS: Extending your legs away from each other.

GAZE: Softly forward at eye level or up to your raised arms.

HOLD: 5 breaths, then release and change legs.

VARIATIONS: Stay on the knee of the back leg if needed and keep your groin raised. Place your hands on blocks for lift if necessary. Place a bolster under your groin for support if necessary.

BENEFITS: Stretches your hamstrings and inner legs; stimulates circulation to the groin and pelvic organs; tones the nerves of the legs and relieves sciatica.

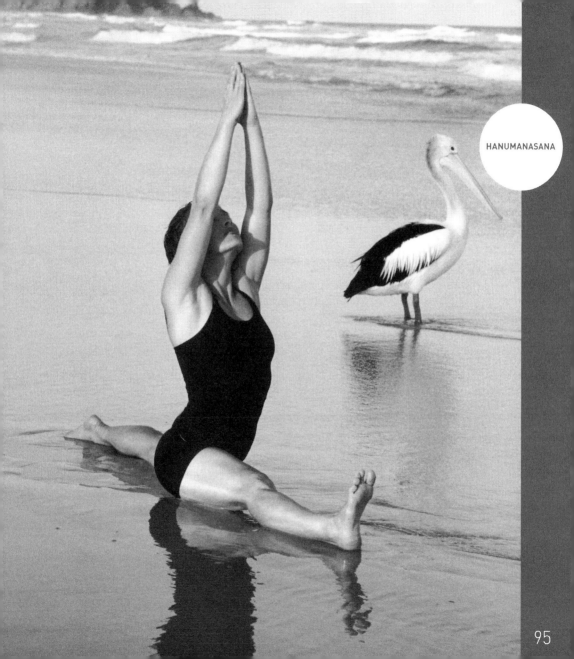

HANUMANASANA

95

SAMAKONASANA

SAMAKONASANA
SAMA – SAME/EVEN; *KONA* – ANGLE

As body and mind melt, your soul strengthens to remain firm and relaxed in this beautifully powerful posture.

POSITIONING: Stand upright, then slowly slide your feet wide apart until your groin rests on the floor and your legs are fully extended out to the sides creating a strong, straight line. Turn your feet upright and flex your toes. Place your palms together in front of your heart center, drop your shoulders, open your chest and lengthen up and out from your hips (as shown in main photo). To go deeper into the opening, drop your chest to the floor, extending your arms and legs out to the side; roll the pelvis forward so your hips and feet are in line, turning your feet down to rest on the floor. Soften the groin to the floor sliding your feet away and look forward (inset photo).

FOCUS: Softening the groin and inner leg muscles.

GAZE: Softly ahead at eye level.

BREATHING: Deep, full breaths.

HOLD: 5–10 breaths. To release, place your hands on the floor in front of you and walk your feet in and back up to standing.

VARIATION: Place your palms on the floor and lift your groin, focusing on softening toward the floor with the breath.

BENEFITS: Tones the nerves of your legs; stretches your legs and hips; stimulates blood flow to your pelvic organs; relieves sciatica.

EKA PADA SIRSASANA
EKA – ONE; *PADA* – LEG/FOOT; *SIRSA* – HEAD

A strong sense of adventure and creativity is inherent in this intricate design; practice from stillness to achieve softness and grace.

POSITIONING: Sit on the floor with your legs outstretched in front. Raise your right leg, catching the ankle with your right hand. Extend your right leg upward to stretch the hamstrings, then bring the foot and upper leg behind your head. Roll your shoulders back and bring your leg as far back as possible, working your neck muscles to slide the foot down away from the back of your head. Lift out of your hips and bring your palms together in front of your heart center. Keep your left leg stretched out in front with the toes flexed and keep yourself seated firmly on the floor.

FOCUS: Lengthening your torso upward and drawing your shoulders back to create space for your chest.

GAZE: Softly ahead at eye level.

BREATHING: Slow down the breath for mental stillness.

HOLD: 5 breaths, then release and change legs.

VARIATION: If you cannot bring your leg behind your head, keep stretching the leg upwards, aiming to soften the muscles of the back of the leg and open the hamstrings.

BENEFITS: Stretches your hamstrings; tones the nerves of your legs; strengthens your neck and spinal muscles; stimulates circulation to your abdominal organs.

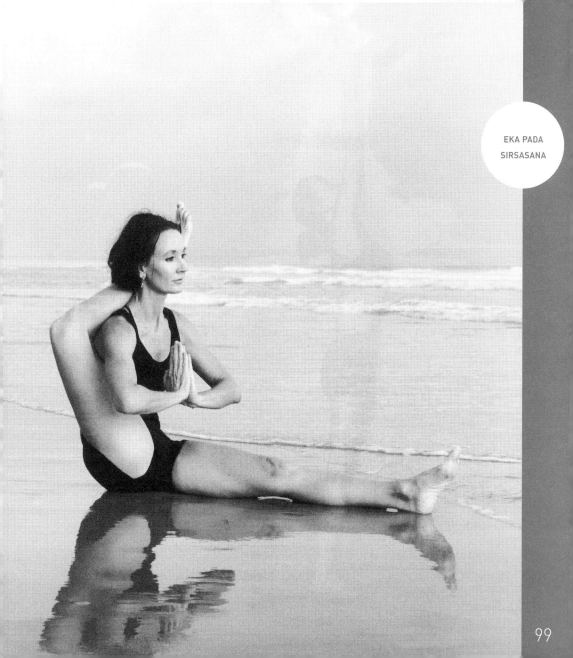

LYING-DOWN POSTURES

When you lie flat on your back or stomach, your nervous system gets
the message to relax, and you can use the conserved energy to lengthen
and strengthen your body with minimal effort or strain. In this way, the supine
and prone postures that follow require little exertion yet are deeply effective in
strengthening and stretching the whole body. Remember, the body often heals and
changes the most in a restful position.

Many of the postures in this section work to tone the core center — the abdominal and lower
back region — which has many benefits. A strong abdominal wall and lower back provide your
spine and hips with good support when you walk and move about, your posture improves and
your abdominal organs have somewhere to rest safely. It makes sense to be strong in your
center; with this strong core, you can move your entire body with ease and minimal effort.

When practicing these inner and outer strength-building postures, always do so with
breath-awareness and care. Only do what feels right and do not extend beyond a
sensible pain threshold. Take care not to strain your back or abdominal muscles,
and protect your lower back by keeping your knees bent whenever needed.
Avoid doing these lying-down postures if you have back or neck
problems, or during the first three days of the menstrual cycle.
If you are pregnant, consult a yoga teacher who
specializes in prenatal postures for safe
modifications.

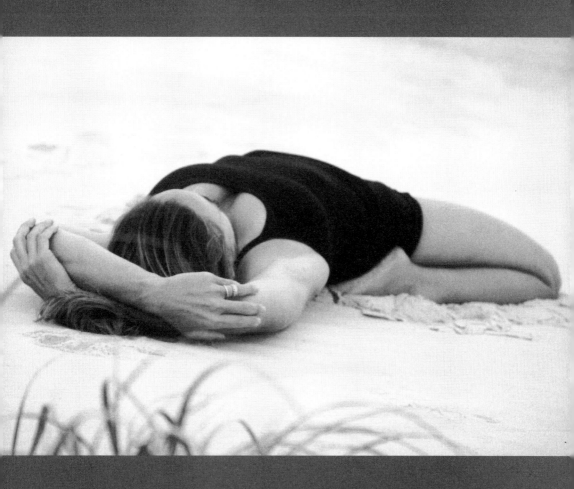

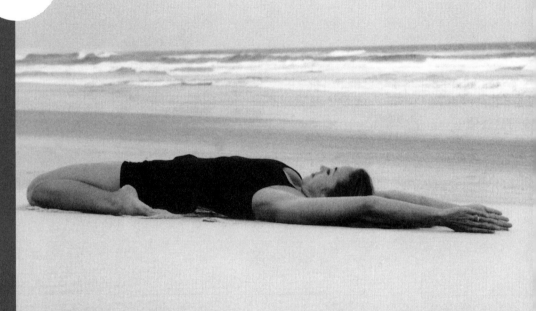

SUPTA VIRASANA
SUPTA – SUPINE; *VIRA* – INDIAN HERO

This wonderful therapeutic posture relieves indigestion so practice it
when you have overeaten or to relieve stomach tension.

POSITIONING: Kneel on the floor with your knees together and your
buttocks raised. Turn your calves out and tuck your tailbone under as you
slowly sink down to rest your buttocks on the floor between your heels, the top
of your feet in contact with the floor. Place your hands on the soles of your feet
and lift your buttocks off the floor, tucking your tail bone under. Looking forward,
slowly start to lower yourself to the floor until you are lying flat on your back
between the heels of your feet. Lengthen out of your lower back and try to tuck
under your tail bone even more to flatten your back to the floor. Keeping your chin
tucked in, inhale to extend your arms over your head, shoulder-width apart. Extend
out through your fingertips, keeping your arms active and lengthening your whole
torso out from your hips.

FOCUS: Keeping your knees pressing down and together and your outer
thighs rolling in; flattening the whole front of your body from your thighs to your
upper chest.

GAZE: At the tip of your nose.

BREATHING: Long, slow inhalations to expand your chest; long, slow
exhalations, drawing your navel back to your spine.

HOLD: 10–25 breaths, then inhale to release up.

VARIATIONS: Lie back over a bolster placed vertically to support your
whole spine and head to relieve back tension. Place padding under
your knees to prevent back strain if needed.

BENEFITS: Stretches the whole front of your torso, hips and knees;
tones your stomach and digestive system; stimulates circulation
to the abdominal organs.

ARCHED SUPTA VIRASANA
SUPTA – SUPINE; *VIRA* – INDIAN HERO

Open your heart and lungs, release blocks and pains, and free yourself for a new lease on life and love.

POSITIONING: From *Supta Virasana* (pages 102–103), place your hands on the soles of your feet and drop the crown of your head back toward the floor, bending your elbows and moving your chest forward, puffing it out. Lengthen up out of your lower back to get more stretch through your front. Rest your elbows to the floor and allow your head to drop back (as shown in top photo). If you cannot sit in *Virasana* bent-leg position, keep your legs extended straight (bottom photo).

FOCUS: Keeping your knees down and together; stretching open your chest.

GAZE: At the tip of your nose.

BREATHING: Deep, full breaths.

HOLD: 5 breaths, then inhale to release up, pressing your hands to your feet.

BENEFITS: Opens your chest, heart, respiratory muscles and shoulders; strengthens your back; stimulates your nervous system; stretches the front of your hips and knees.

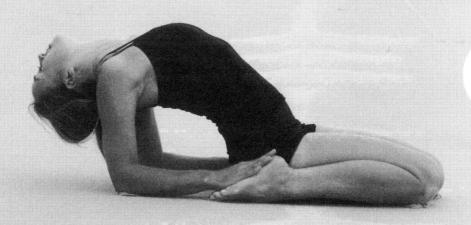

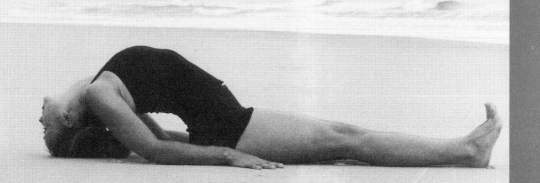

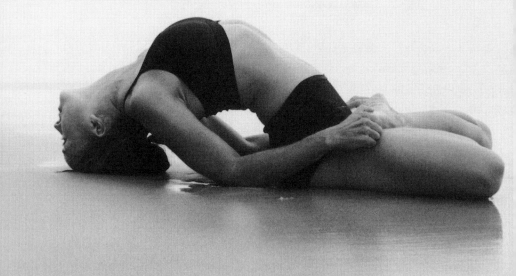

MATSYASANA
MATSYA – FISH

Open your throat fully to enhance communication skills, the power of speech and self-love.

POSITIONING: Sit on the floor with your legs extended in front. Raise your right leg and roll the thigh outward as you place your right foot on the left upper thigh. Let your right knee sink to the floor. Raise your left leg and place your left foot on the right upper thigh. Allow both knees to rest on the floor with your hips opening outward. Keep your spine extending upward from your pelvic base. Drop onto your back, tucking your head under so that your throat opens, and rest the crown of your head on the floor. Reach for your feet with your hands, grabbing them and pressing your elbows to the floor to get a deeper arch in the back and lift your chest out further.

FOCUS: Keeping both knees pressing down. Using your arms as levers to get more lift.

GAZE: Focus on the third-eye point between your eyebrows.

BREATHING: Long, slow even breaths through your nose.

HOLD: 5 breaths, then inhale to release.

BENEFITS: Stretches your abdominal wall and organs; opens your chest, heart, lungs, throat and hips; tones your back and spinal cord; stretches your knees.

DWI PADA SIRSASANA
DWI – TWO; *PADA* – LEG/FOOT; *SIRSA* – HEAD

Wrapped up safe in your own embrace, find yourself at peace with where you are, with what is.

POSITIONING: Sit on the floor with your legs extended in front. Raise your right leg, catching the ankle with both hands. Extend your right leg upright, stretching the hamstrings, then take the foot and upper leg behind your head to rest behind your neck. When you have your balance, lie down on your back, ensuring your right leg is locked in behind your head. Raise your left leg and place it behind your head over your right leg. Slide the feet down further to lock them in and point your toes away. Press your shoulders back to make more room for the front of your torso, and drop your buttocks and lower back to the floor. Bring the palms of your hands together in prayer position in front of your heart center.

FOCUS: Using your neck muscles to keep your legs back.

GAZE: Softly and serenely forward.

BREATHING: Soft and even breaths.

HOLD: 5–10 breaths, then release and rest.

BENEFITS: Stretches your leg, spine and neck muscles; tones the nerves of your legs.

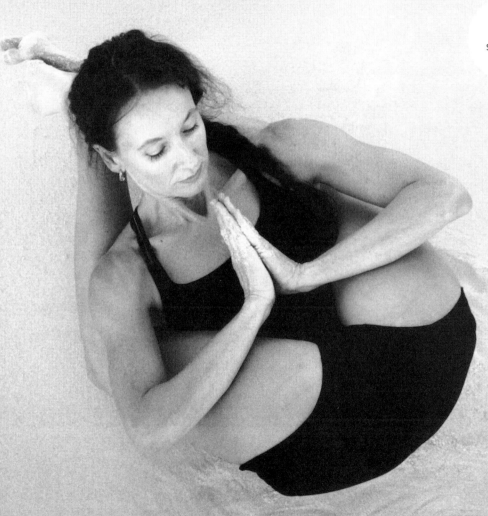

BACKWARD-BENDING POSTURES

The exotically shaped backward-bending postures have beauty, strength, endurance and
balance to give. They evoke feelings of openness, freedom and joy. From a relatively simple
upward bend that frees the muscles of the chest to a dynamic full-body curl that reaches deep into
the muscles that power your heart, backward bends come in many variations to challenge bodies of all
strengths and flexibility.

Arching back counteracts the spine's natural tendency to compress and limit mobility with age. Backward
bends promote good health, good posture and flexibility of body and mind. Doing them regularly keeps the
chest open and the circulation flowing freely to the heart and lungs, oxygenating the whole body. They also
activate the nervous system, awakening the mind, and generate heat throughout the body, stimulating
metabolism, promoting weight loss and encouraging the body's natural cleansing processes.

Bending back and opening the chest also unlocks the spirit within. Practicing these postures takes you along
previously untraveled paths, challenging you to overcome fear and frustration, teaching you to move with ease
and grace, and to live with an open heart and a passion for life and love.

Working with the breath is the key to being calm and open in a backward bend. Use the inhalation to
lengthen out of your lower back and all the way along the spine. Use the exhalation to soften and
release deeper into the posture.

Avoid backward bending if you have back problems, or speak with a remedial yoga teacher for
modifications and props that are suitable for you. It is not advisable to practice strenuous
backward-bending postures while you are menstruating, if you are new to yoga,
while you are pregnant, or if you have a weak heart or high blood pressure.

Always counterbalance these backward arching postures with
forward bends to lengthen and straighten your spine
and calm the nervous system.

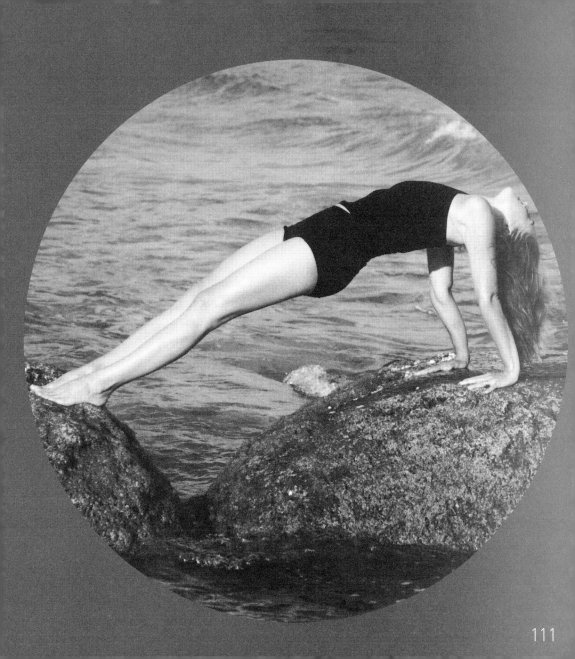

111

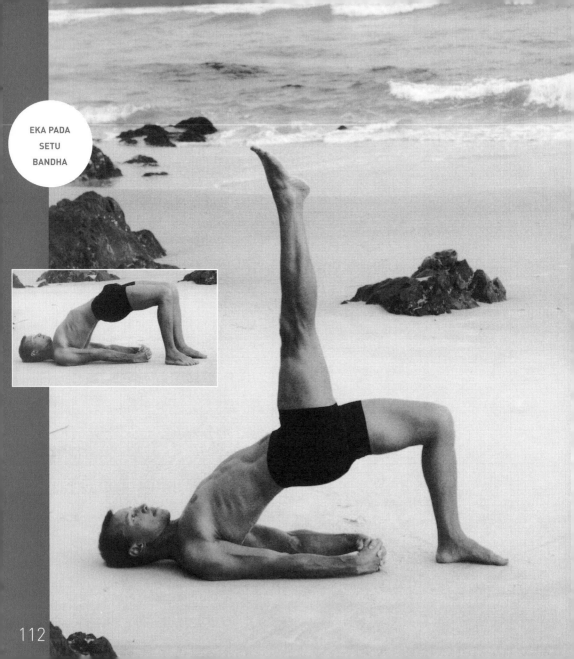

EKA PADA
SETU
BANDHA

EKA PADA SETU BANDHA
EKA – ONE; *PADA* – LEG/FOOT; *SETU* – BRIDGE;
BANDHA – FORMATION

A stunning formation that helps develop a strong back and mind and the ability to find stillness within even through life's challenges.

POSITIONING: Lie flat on your back on the floor with your chin tucked in to your neck. Bend your knees and place your feet close to your buttocks, hip-width apart, with your arms extending toward your feet. Press your arms, wrists and palms to the floor. Inhale to roll your pelvis, then your lower, middle and upper back off the floor so you are resting on the top of your shoulders. Interlock your fingers underneath your raised back, extending your arms on the floor. Lift your pubic bone high and keep your knees hip-width apart (as shown in inset photo). Inhale to raise your right leg straight up into the air to create a vertical line, your toes pointing upward (main photo). At the same time, drop your right hip so that it remains at the same level as the left. Press the big-toe side of your left foot firmly into the floor to activate your inner-leg muscles.

FOCUS: Extending your leg high, keeping your back arched and chest open.

GAZE: At the foot of the extended leg.

BREATHING: Deep, full breathing.

HOLD: 5 breaths, then release and change sides.

BENEFITS: Strengthens your lower back, abdominal muscles and legs; opens your chest and shoulders; tones the spinal nerves and organs; develops endurance.

URDHVA
DHANURASANA I

URDHVA DHANURASANA I
URDHVA – UPWARDS; *DHANU* – A BOW

Experience lightness and buoyancy as you extend outward and upward
in this dynamic back flexion and help prevent spinal degeneration.

POSITIONING: Lie flat on your back with your legs bent and your feet placed
close to your buttocks, hip-width apart. Tuck your fingers underneath your
shoulders, your elbows pointing up and away from your head. Inhale deeply, then
exhale to lift your buttocks, torso and head off the floor. Extend out through your
arms and legs, pushing upward and away from the floor as high as possible (as
shown in inset photo). Lengthen out of your lower back, lifting your navel high and
moving your chest forward. Lift your pubis and navel area upward and lengthen up
through your legs. Keep the outside edge of your feet parallel and work your inner
leg muscles by pressing the big-toe side of your feet firmly to the floor. Exhale to
raise your right leg high into the air (main photo). Keep your right leg activated and
point your toes away, moving your leg higher and closer to your head with each
breath. Keep your arms lengthened and the lower leg working strongly. Move your
chest forward and your pubis upward.

FOCUS: Lifting up and away from the floor.

GAZE: Softly toward the floor.

BREATHING: Soft, even breaths for stability and calm.

HOLD: 5 breaths, then release the leg down and change sides.

BENEFITS: Softens and stretches the spine, helping prevent shrinking
and degeneration; increases blood flow to your head and brain;
stimulates the nervous system; stimulates metabolism; opens
your heart; helps relieve depression and sluggishness; helps
develop grace.

URDHVA DHANURASANA II
URDHVA – UPWARD; *DHANU* – BOW

Enhance inspiration and openness of chest, heart and lungs in this straight-legged backward bend.

POSITIONING: Lie flat on your back with your legs bent and feet placed close up to your buttocks, hip-width apart. Tuck your fingers underneath your shoulders, your elbows pointing away from your head. Inhale deeply then exhale to lift your buttocks, torso and head off the floor. Extend out through your arms and legs, pushing upward and away from the floor as high as possible. Lengthen out of your lower back, lifting your navel high and moving your chest forward. Lift your pubis and navel area upward and lengthen your legs. Inhale to press your chest forward between your shoulders further and straighten your legs so that the knees are locked and your toes are pressed to the floor; to do this, you may need to walk your feet away from your head a little more. Keep the outside edge of your feet parallel.

FOCUS: Lengthening the whole front of your body; elongating out of your lower back; moving your chest forward.

GAZE: At the tip of your nose.

BREATHING: Deep and focused.

HOLD: 5 breaths, then release and repeat.

BENEFITS: Tones your legs and spine; strengthens your lower back; stretches the abdominal wall; stimulates the nervous system; opens your heart and lungs.

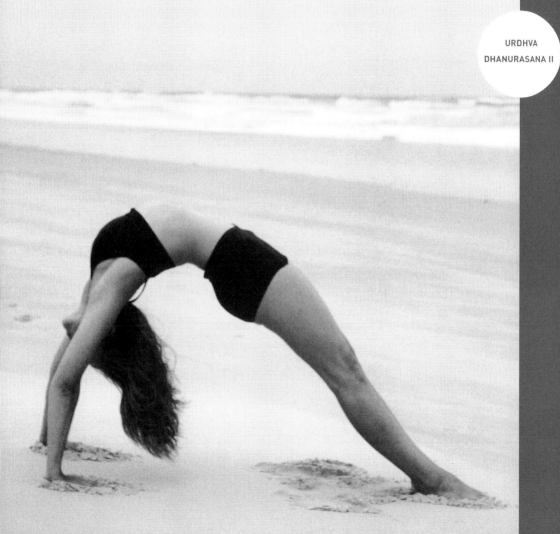

EKA PADA RAJAKAPOTASANA
EKA – ONE; *PADA* – FOOT/LEG;
RAJA – KING; *KAPOTA* – PIGEON

Beauty, strength and grace are yours through practicing this exquisite pose with deep, full breathing for softness and ease.

POSITIONING: Lie on your stomach with your legs extending back. Bring your hands, palms down, beside your torso and lift up. Bend your left leg and slide your left foot forward so that the knee sits behind your left wrist and your left foot rests close in to your groin. Slide your hands next to your hips and lengthen up and out of your lower back, rolling your shoulders back. Put your hands on your hips, drop your head back, and raise your arms over your head, palms together (see inset photo).
Then, bend your right leg and catch the top of your right foot behind your head, first with your right hand and then with both hands. Holding the top of your foot, lift up and out of your lower back. Drawing your foot closer to your head, drop your head back. Puffing your chest forward, move your foot to rest against the back of your head. Keeping your hips parallel to each other, bring your elbows together and pointing upwards, extending the space from the sides of your torso, armpits and through each elbow tip.

FOCUS: Lengthening out of your lower back; softening to open your chest.

GAZE: Focus on the third-eye point between your eyebrows.

BREATHING: Deep, full breaths through your nose for deep opening.

HOLD: 5 breaths, then release and change sides.

VARIATIONS: Use a strap to catch hold of the back leg if you cannot reach your foot. Place a folded blanket under the buttock of your front leg for balance.

BENEFITS: Tones your spine and creates a supple back; opens your chest, heart and respiratory muscles; strengthens your legs.

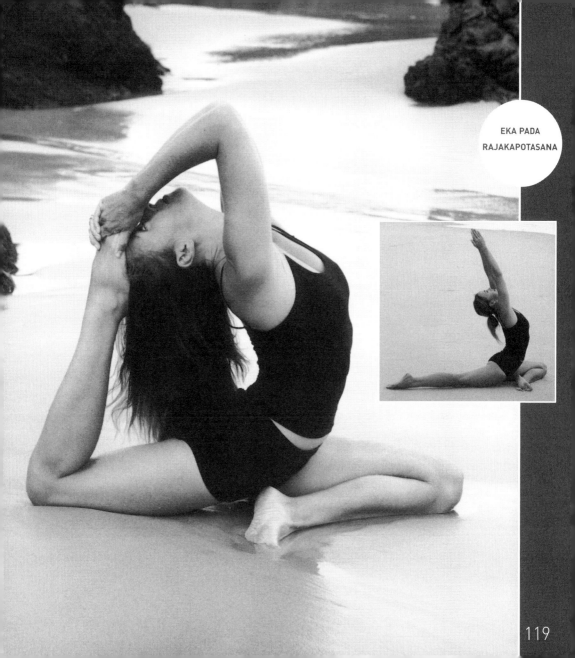

EKA PADA
RAJAKAPOTASANA

119

NATARAJASANA

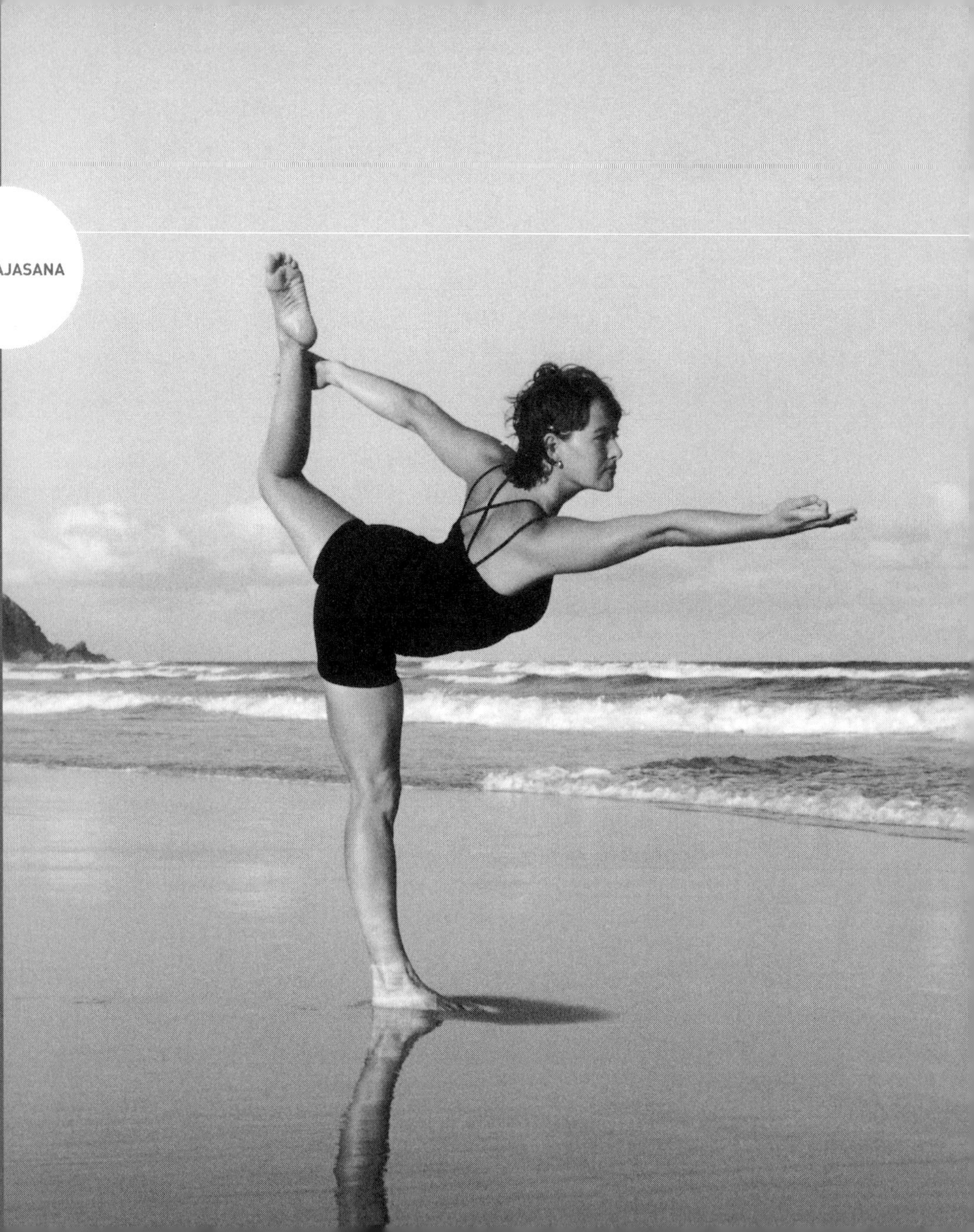

NATARAJASANA
NATA – DANCER; *RAJA* – KING

Live the beauty and grace of the dance in this uplifting pose.

POSITIONING: Stand upright and extend your right arm straight out in front. Bend your left knee and lift your leg to the back, grasping your left ankle at the front. Roll your arm around so that the elbow faces upward. Lift your leg so that the left thigh is parallel with the ground. Puff your chest out as you lift up through your spine. Extend the back leg up high.

FOCUS: Deepening the flexion in your spine; locking the standing leg.

GAZE: Softly ahead.

BREATHING: Use the breath to move deeper into the posture.

HOLD: 5 breaths, then release and change sides.

VARIATION: Use a strap around the raised foot if you cannot reach your foot with your hand.

BENEFITS: Opens your chest, heart and lungs; tones your spine and spinal nerves; strengthens your legs; helps develop deep, full breathing, balance and coordination.

KAPOTASANA
KAPOTA – PIGEON

As your whole body reverses in this pose, your spine will undergo total
rejuvenation and renewal that will be reflected in the way you experience your life.

POSITIONING: From *Supta Virasana* (pages 102–103), tuck your fingers
underneath your shoulders and, pressing your palms to the floor, inhale to lift your
head, chest, buttocks and upper legs off the floor. Rest in this position for a breath
and then, keeping your head dropped back, begin to walk your hands, one at
a time, in towards your feet until you can grasp your toes or heels. Lift up through
your torso and lengthen out of your lower back. Keep lifting your hips as you bring
your chest forward. Keep your inner legs active and your tail bone tucking under.

FOCUS: Puffing your chest forward; rolling the outer thighs in.

GAZE: At the tip of your nose.

BREATHING: Soften with the breath to find calmness in the pose.

HOLD: 5 breaths, then release and rest.

BENEFITS: Radically bends your spine for flexibility and suppleness;
stimulates your nervous system; increases blood flow to your pelvic region;
stretches your abdominal area.

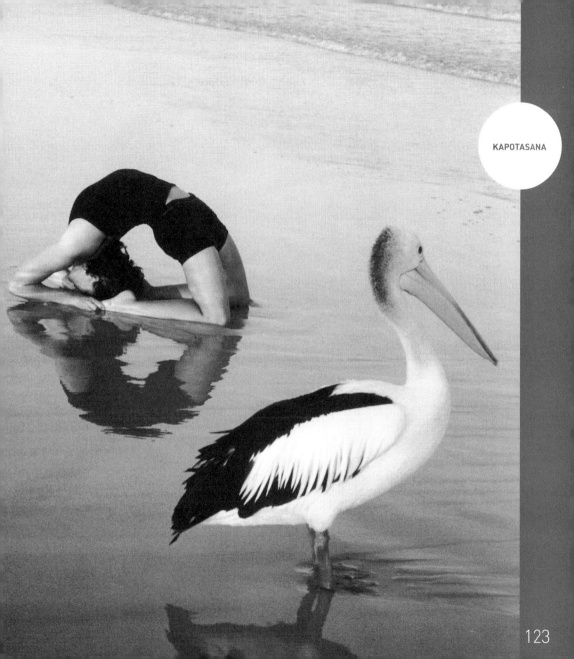

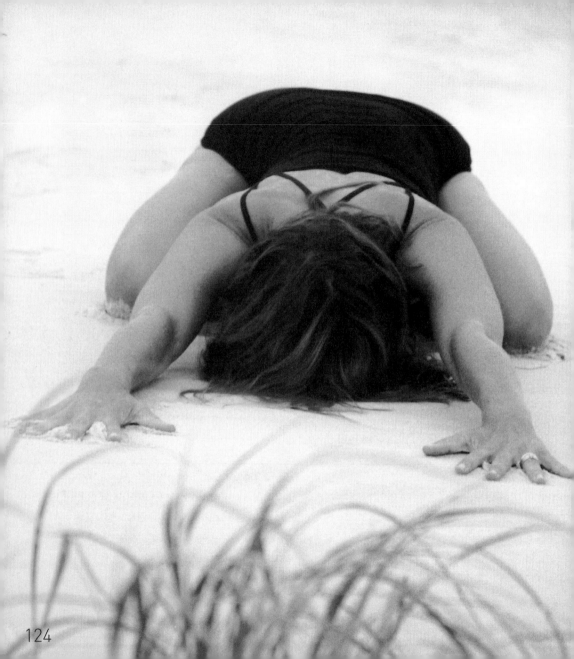

FORWARD-BENDING POSTURES

Foster a deep inner connection by sinking into a restful forward-bending posture. As your body reclines forward and down, your metabolism slows, creating a cooling effect, your nervous system relaxes and your mind calms. Turning inward is not always easy, particularly if your day-to-day routine requires a lot of outward focus. But you can balance your extroverted life with these introverted postures and create harmony of body and mind. If resistance or frustration arises in your yoga practice or in life, take a deep breath and let go completely, allowing your mind to relax and your body to yield.

Physically, the forward-bending postures have many benefits, such as opening your hamstrings, loosening a tight back or inner leg muscles, strengthening the front of your legs and knees, toning your abdominal area and opening your chest and shoulders.

Emotionally, a forward bend helps develop self-awareness and the ability to connect with your inner self. From this point of inner connection, truth and real-ness with your self and others is enhanced.

Practice a forward-bending posture following a backward bend to release any holding in the muscles of the back and legs, or whenever you need to turn inward, away from the external world, to find quiet. The forward bends are a retreat in themselves.

Use a strap around your feet to lengthen forward if you cannot reach your feet with your hands. Sitting on the edge of a folded blanket also helps tilt your pelvis forward and increases forward lengthening.

Work in the postures intelligently with deep, full breathing through your nose. As you lengthen forward, always do so from the front of your torso and not from your lower lumbar spine. Use the inhalation to lengthen from the front, lifting the skin on the front of your torso, belly and chest. Use the exhalation to soften and release downward.

Avoid strenuous forward-bending postures if you have back problems and seek modifications from a remedial yoga teacher if necessary.

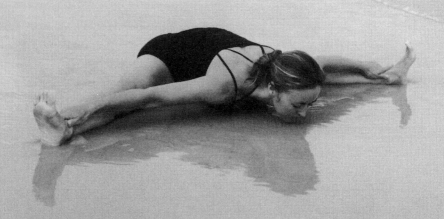

UPAVISTHA KONASANA
UPAVISTHA – SEATED; *KONA* – ANGLE

Stretch your body, mind and spirit toward a happier and healthier state of being in this widening position.

POSITIONING: Sit on the floor and extend your legs out wide to the sides with your feet upright. Lengthen out through the back of your legs, pressing the back of your knees down and pressing out through the balls and heels of your feet. Flex your toes back toward your hips. Holding your big toes or the outside edge of your feet, inhale to lengthen from the front of your torso. Exhale to bring your lower abdomen, chest and chin to the floor. Keep your buttocks on the floor, your thighs rolling back and your feet upright.

FOCUS: Softening the inner leg muscles and hamstrings; lengthening from the front.

GAZE: Softly forward and down.

BREATHING: Deep, full breaths through your nose.

HOLD: 10 breaths or for as long as comfortable.

VARIATION: Sit on the edge of 2–3 folded blankets for comfort and to assist forward tilting.

BENEFITS: Opens your hips and inner leg muscles; stretches the muscles of the back of your legs; strengthens the front of your legs; stimulates blood flow to your pelvic organs.

KURMASANA
KURMA – TORTOISE

Turn your back on the external world, deepen your inward journey and find that restful space where there is just you and the breath.

POSITIONING: Sit on the floor with your legs extended in front of you about 3 feet apart. Inhale to lengthen and extend forward. Slide your arms under your legs, bringing your shoulders under your knees. Soften your torso to the floor and extend through the ball and heels of your feet, and flex your toes back. Press the back of your knees to the floor and lock your legs. Keep lengthening the front of your torso along the floor, softening deeper into the inner legs and hamstrings. Bring your forehead or chin to the floor.

FOCUS: Softening in the inner legs; extending your arms and legs; pressing the backs of your knees down.

GAZE: Softly at the tip of your nose.

BREATHING: Listen to the soft sound of your breath.

BENEFITS: Opens your inner leg, hip and groin muscles; stimulates blood flow to nourish your pelvic organs; tones your legs; helps develop deep inner calm.

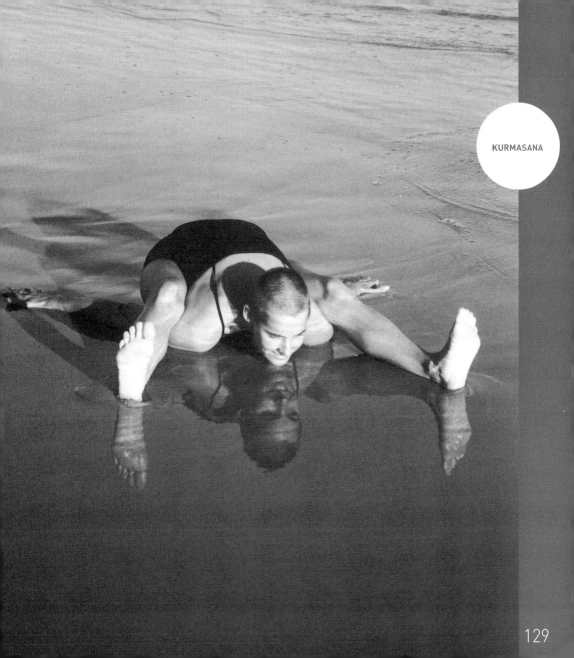

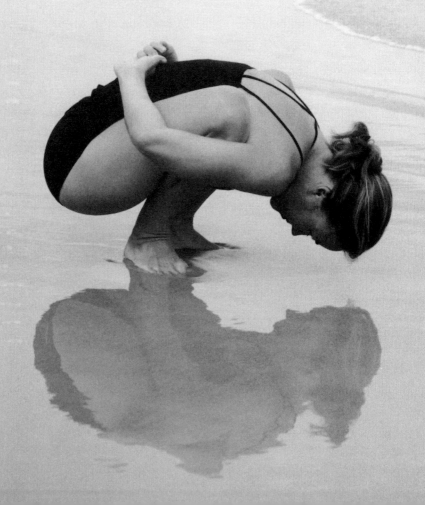

MALASANA
MALA – NOOSE

This delicate loop, which refines your inner balance and cultivates calmness, requires firmness, poise and focused intention.

POSITIONING: Squat with your heels together, feet turned out and knees wide apart. Inhale to lengthen from the front of your torso, stretching your torso and arms through your knees. Exhale to wrap your arms around your back, interlocking your fingers wherever you can reach in the lower back area. Extend from your front as far as possible. When you have found your full position, drop your head forward.

FOCUS: Pressing your heels to the floor and maintaining balance.

GAZE: At the tip of your nose.

BREATHING: Slow, even breaths through your nose.

VARIATIONS: Place a folded blanket underneath your heels for support. Use a strap to catch your hands behind you for balance. If needed, keep your hands outstretched in front.

BENEFITS: Tones your legs; opens your ankles and hips; stimulates blood flow to your pelvic region and abdominal organs; stretches your back.

SKANDASANA
SKANDA – WAR GOD

This complicated *asana* reflects the intricacies of your being and your ability to resist and conquer.

POSITIONING: From *Eka Pada Sirsasana* (pages 98–99) exhale to extend your torso forward and down along your outstretched leg, catching the foot or turning your palms out around the foot and interlocking your fingers. Rest your chin on your knee or shinbone and gaze toward the foot of your extended leg. Keep your back and neck strong, resisting from allowing the foot to collapse into your head. Align your torso so that you lie straight along the extended leg.

FOCUS: Keeping your head slightly tilted upward to support and stabilize the leg behind your head.

GAZE: Toward the foot of your extended leg.

BREATHING: Slowly.

VARIATION: Place your hands on the floor wherever needed for balance and support.

BENEFITS: Strengthens your upper back and neck muscles; invigorates your immune system; stretches your hamstrings; stimulates your digestive system; softens your legs.

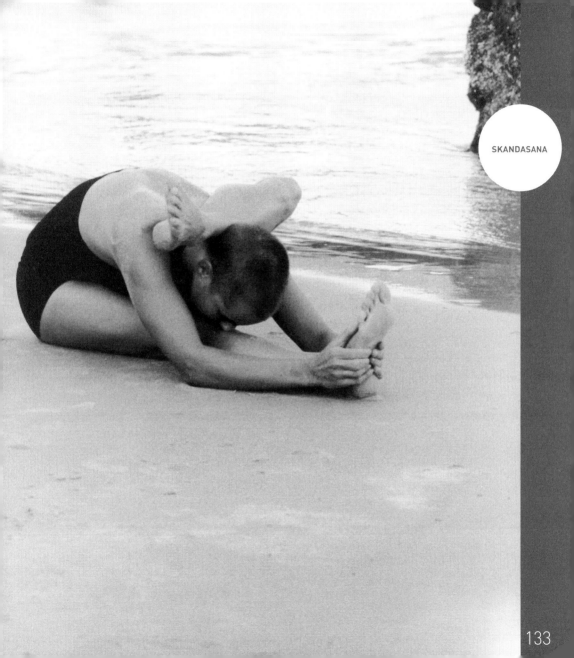

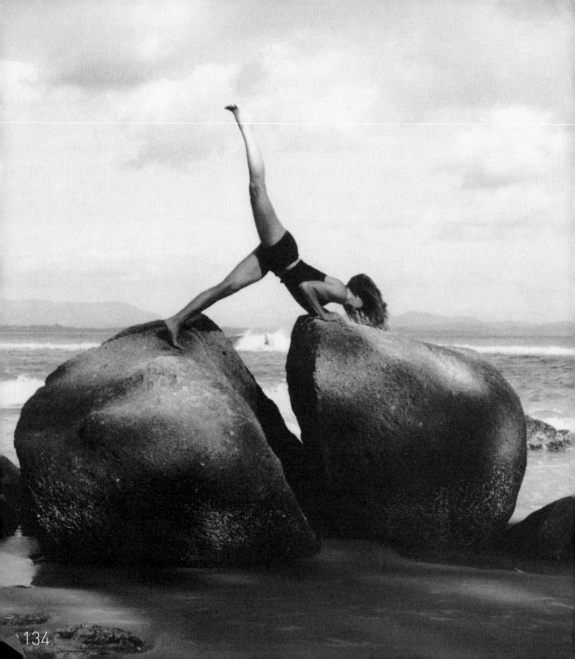

INVERTED POSTURES

Inversions offer the unique experience of being in the opposite position from the way you spend most of your life – head-down rather than standing, sitting and lying. When you put yourself head first, you challenge your regular perspective of life and view the world in reverse. For the sake of lightness of being and openness of mind, it makes good creative sense to get upside-down on a regular basis.

Turning upside-down stimulates the flow of oxygenated blood, which assists in nourishment, cell regeneration and waste elimination. It also increases blood flow to the brain, relieving mental fatigue and promoting clear thinking and a good memory. Inverted postures also relieve tiredness, cleanse and tone your body and soothe aching legs and feet. Defying gravity's natural downward pull, inverted postures help to reverse the aging process, toning your skin and soft tissue, and giving a youthful oxygenated glow from the inside out. These playful, if often intricate, postures come in many forms and can be explored from the head, hands or forearms. Your ability to do them will improve with practice, as your balance, coordination and strength develop. You need to be focused to maintain the postures and to move in and out of them with ease. The breath is the key to calmness and endurance in these positions, as well as the ability to direct energy through your whole body for even weight distribution and balance. With practice, you will become aware of your whole body working in unison and you will become more creative than ever, discovering limitless potential in life's journey.

It is best to learn the following postures with an experienced yoga teacher. Being shown the correct way to work in such postures will help to avoid injury and deepen your understanding and experience of them. Do not practice inversions if your neck is sore, if you are menstruating, or if you have high blood pressure, a weak heart or brain problems. If you are pregnant, consult a prenatal yoga teacher for safe modifications. Use props to assist with support and comfort, such as a wall to lean against, folded blankets to support your neck and a strap tied above your elbows, shoulder-width apart, to prevent your arms from splaying out.

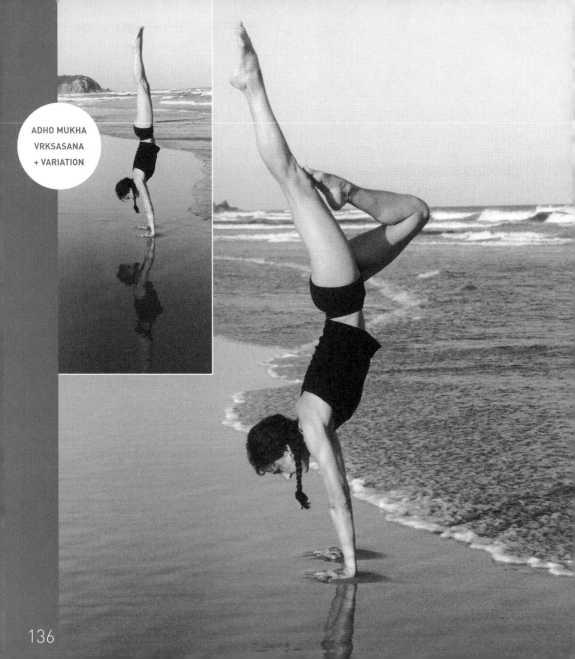

ADHO MUKHA
VRKSASANA
+ VARIATION

136

ADHO MUKHA VRKSASANA

+ VARIATION
ADHO – DOWN; *MUKHA* – FACE;
VRKSA – TREE

Balance on your palms to allow your body and mind to creatively unite and to achieve perfect equilibrium.

POSITIONING: Stand upright then lean down and place the palms of your hands flat on the floor in front of your feet. Spread your fingers wide and look down between your hands at the floor. Walk your feet in until your shoulders are above your hands. Lengthen up through your arms, activating your arm muscles. Get in contact with your abdominal muscles and contract them. Bring your feet together and inhale to bend your knees and hop up, extending your legs up in a full handstand. Use your abdominal muscles to lift and continue to look down between your hands. Lengthen up through your arms and legs, keeping your tail bone tucked under slightly and your whole body in a straight line. Lock your legs, keeping your feet together in this first position (as shown in inset photo). Bend your right leg and slide your right foot down to rest on your left knee. Hold this second position (main photo) then release and change legs.

FOCUS: Developing an awareness of your core center.

GAZE: Between your hands at the floor.

BREATHING: Inhale to kick up, then normal breathing. Exhale to come down.

HOLD: For as long as possible; exhale down with your feet together and your legs straight, bending at the hips and using your abdominal muscles for control.

VARIATION: Use a wall for support; place your hands one hand-distance back from the wall and kick up one leg at a time.

BENEFITS: Develops a strong upper body; stimulates circulation to your head and brain; encourages internal cleansing; tones your skin; stimulates your nervous system.

PADMA PINCA MAYURASANA
PADMA – LOTUS; *PINCA* – TAIL FEATHER;
MAYURA – PEACOCK

Use the steadiness and ease found in this posture to move with the breath further into creativity and exploration.

POSITIONING: Kneel with your hands and elbows on the floor. Create a right angle with your forearms along the floor, your upper arms lifting. Spread your fingers wide and press your palms and wrists firmly to the floor. Keep your hands and elbows shoulder-width apart. Look at the floor between your thumbs as you lift your head upward. Step your feet back, lifting your buttocks and hips, and straightening your legs. Exhale to kick your legs up, one at a time. Bring your feet and legs together and lengthen up and away from your forearms. Lift your shoulders and press your wrists firmly to the ground. This is the first position, *Pinca Mayurasana* (as shown in inset photo). Bring your left foot to rest on top of your right thigh, then flick your right foot to cross over the left and rest on top of your left upper thigh. Come into full *Padmasana* position (main photo), bringing your knees back to open your hips more. Keep lifting in your shoulders and chest.

FOCUS: Lifting up through your upper arms, shoulders and chest.

GAZE: Between your hands at the floor.

BREATHING: Deep, full breaths through your nose.

HOLD: For as long as possible, then release, change leg positions and repeat.

VARIATIONS: Tie a strap above your elbows, shoulder-width apart, to keep your arms apart. Place a block between the thumbs and forefingers of each hand to keep your hands shoulder-width apart.

BENEFITS: Strengthens your upper arms, shoulders, chest and back; stretches your legs and knees; increases blood flow to your pelvic organs; stimulates circulation to your head and brain.

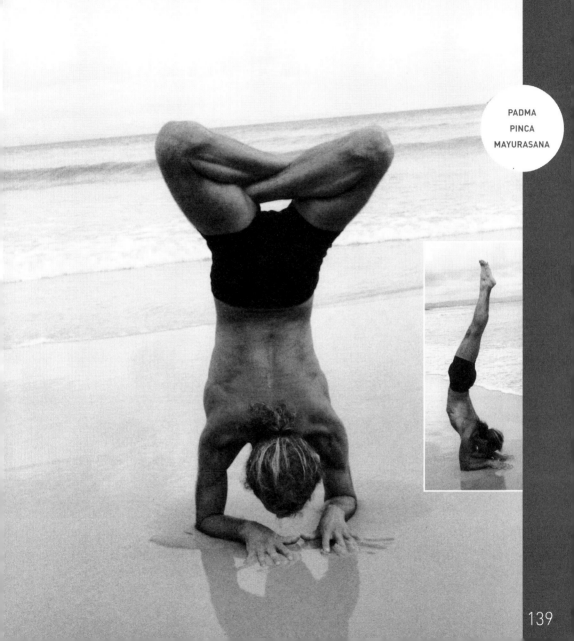

PADMA
PINCA
MAYURASANA

139

VRSCHIKASANA

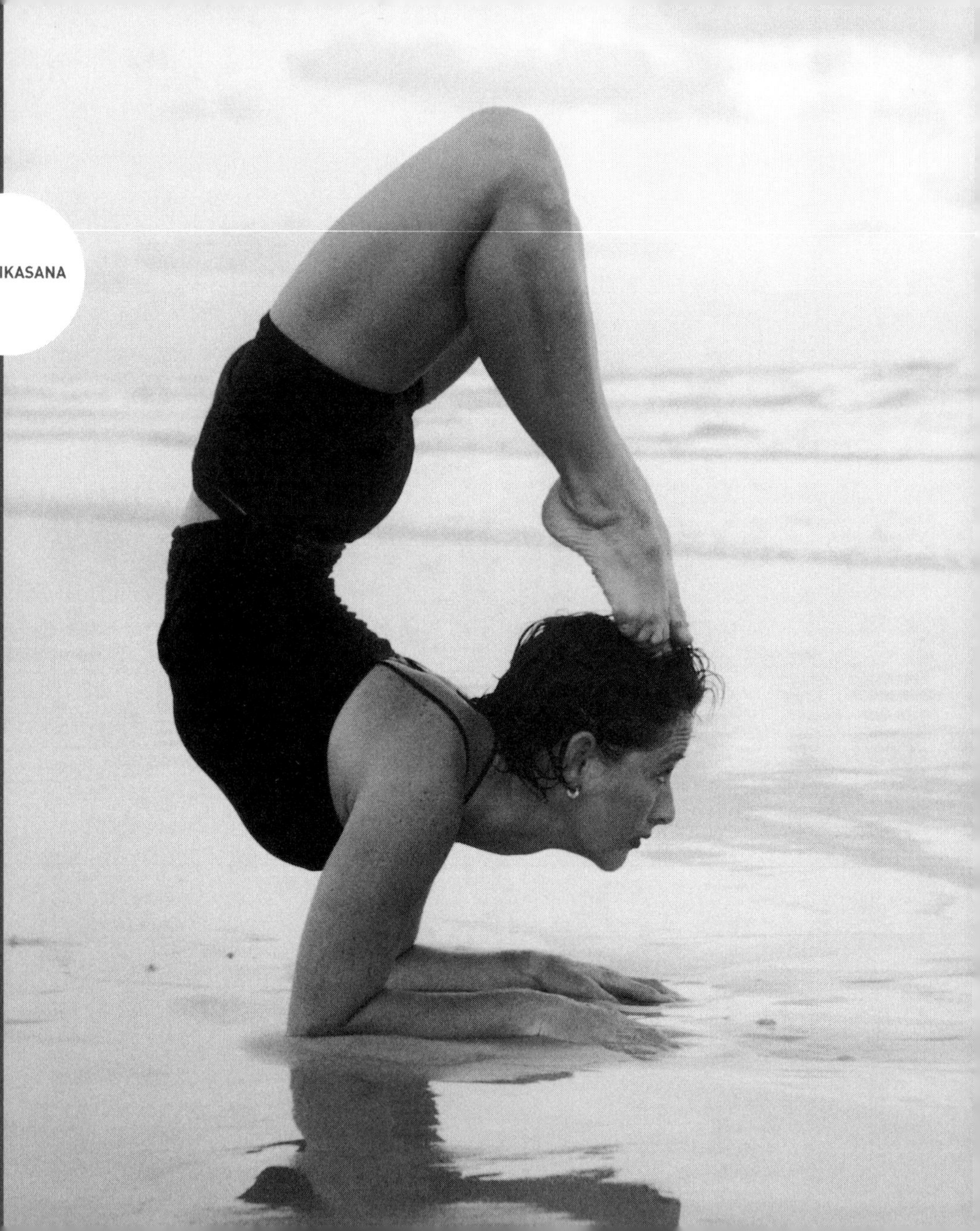

VRSCHIKASANA
VRSCHIKA – SCORPION

A beautifully creative form that will deeply relax your mind and subdue the ego. Practice with soft breath and body.

POSITIONING: From *Padma Pinca Mayurasana* (pages 138–139), keep looking between your hands at the ground and lengthen up through your upper arms and legs. Bend your knees and start to drop your feet behind you toward your back, at the same time lifting out of your lower back and moving your chest forward. Lift your head high and look up toward your descending feet. Arch your back deeply as you continue to bend your legs and drop your feet down to rest on or near your head, looking forward. Your bent legs and torso will create a circle with your feet and head, sealing the form.

FOCUS: Softening your lower back with the breath; puffing your chest forward and straightening your arms.

GAZE: Focus on the third eye point between your eyebrows.

BREATHING: Soften the breath.

HOLD: For as long as comfortable.

BENEFITS: Tones your back and spinal nerves; stretches your abdominal muscles and organs; strengthens your arms, shoulders and chest; tones your heart and lungs; stimulates blood flow to your brain.

KONA SIRSASANA
KONA – ANGLE; *SIRSA* – HEAD

Open your legs wide and experiment with weight distribution, balance, strength and finding lightness and relaxation upside-down.

POSITIONING: From kneeling, bend forward and rest the crown of your head on the floor. Place the little-finger side of your forearms on the floor on either side of your head and interlock your fingers around the back of your head, your palms opening out. Your wrists, little fingers and the side of your forearms should be resting on the floor, and your open palms cupping the back of your head. With the crown of your head on the floor walk your feet in, buttocks and hips lifting high and legs locked. Inhale to extend your legs upright above your head, either one at a time or both together, and lengthen upward. Lift your upper arms and shoulders, chest and the sides of your torso, your pubic bone and legs (as shown in inset photo). Bring your legs wide apart, pointing through your legs and feet. Drop your feet closer toward

the floor as your inner legs and groin open (main photo). Draw your navel back to your spine for core-center support. Keep the muscles of your neck and face relaxed.

FOCUS: Extending out through your legs. Keeping your head lightly on the floor.

GAZE: Softly ahead.

BREATHING: Soft, even breathing to maintain balance.

HOLD: 5 breaths, then return your legs upright to center and repeat twice.

VARIATION: Place a folded blanket under your head for comfort.

BENEFITS: Stretches your inner leg and groin muscles; stimulates blood flow to your pelvic organs, head and brain; promotes internal cleansing; rests your heart; relaxes your nervous system; strengthens your arms and upper torso.

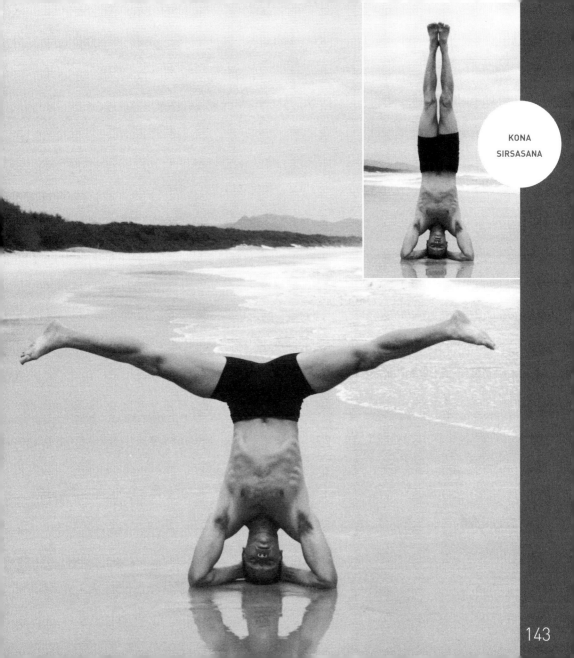

KONA
SIRSASANA

143

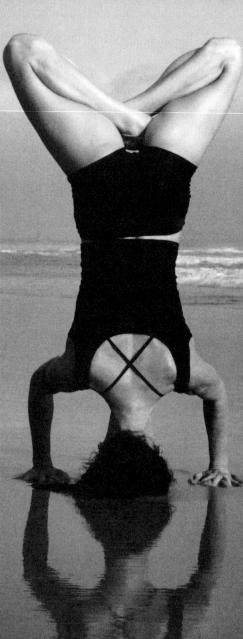

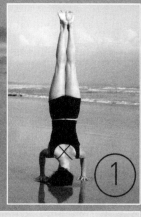

①

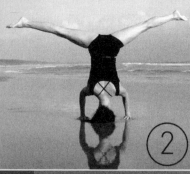

②

③

144

SALAMBA SIRSASANA II
SEQUENCE
SALAMBA – SUPPORTED; *SIRSA* – HEAD

When your body is upside-down and well supported, the potential for growth and creativity expands.

POSITIONING: From kneeling, place the crown of your head on the floor. Lean your torso forward over your head and place the palms of your hands about a foot away from the front of your face, your fingers facing in and your elbows bent to create a right angle with each arm. Center your body weight evenly between the three points of your two hands and the top of your head. Bring your legs up above your head, either together or one at a time. Focus on centering your body weight and extend upwards, lifting through your shoulders, chest, back, hips and legs. Bring your feet together and activate your leg muscles (photo 1). Hold here for 5–10 breaths. Next spread your legs wide apart (photo 2), pointing your toes away and stretching through your inner leg and groin muscles. Hold here for 5 breaths. Then bring your legs back upright with your feet together. Flick your right foot down to rest on top of your left thigh, then flick your left foot to cross over the right and rest on top of your right upper thigh. Come into full *Padmasana* position (photo 3), bringing your knees back to open your hips more. Maintain the lift in your shoulders and chest. Keep the pressure on your head light; don't strain your neck.

FOCUS: Keeping lifted out from your arms and head; keeping your arms at right angles and your elbows shoulder-width apart.

GAZE: Softly ahead.

BREATHING: Slowly for deep relaxation and calm.

HOLD: 10 breaths.

VARIATION: Rest your head on two folded blankets and slide your fingers underneath the blankets.

BENEFITS: Stretches your hips and knees; stimulates blood flow to your pelvis, head and brain; promotes internal cleansing; rests your heart; relaxes your nervous system; strengthens your arms and upper torso; tones your legs.

EKA PADA SARVANGASANA
EKA – ONE; *PADA* – LEG;
SARVANGA – WHOLE BODY

Known as the queen of postures, the shoulder stand is practiced for its therapeutic benefits on the hormonal system and the whole body.

POSITIONING: Lie flat on your back. Lift your legs and roll them over your head. Bring your palms to rest on your back, your elbows and upper arms pressing to the floor. Position your elbows shoulder-width apart and spread your fingers wide on your back to get maximum contact with the skin. Supporting yourself on your head, shoulders, elbows and palms, raise your legs up to a vertical position, making a vertical line from your shoulders out through your feet. Move your palms closer up toward your shoulders and roll onto the top of your shoulders to get more lift. Lengthen up through your back, hips and legs. Draw your navel to your spine and tuck your tailbone under. Keep your feet together and your leg muscles activated. Tuck in your chin and rest the back of your head comfortably on the floor. This is the first position, *Salamba Sarvangasana* (as shown in inset photo). Keep your left leg extending upward as you release your right foot down to the floor in front of your head (main photo). Hold here for 5 breaths, then bring your right leg up and the left foot down for 5 breaths.

FOCUS: Supporting your body with your shoulders and arms; lengthening upward.

GAZE: Softly at your chest.

BREATHING: Focus on the soft airflow through your nostrils.

HOLD: 5 breaths in the first position, and 5 breaths with each leg raised.

VARIATION: Before coming up, elevate your upper back and shoulders on 2–3 neatly folded blankets, your head on the floor, to allow space for your neck to lengthen when you are upright.

BENEFITS: Increases circulation to your glands; calms your nervous system. Helps relieve headaches; rests your heart and lungs; increases the blood flow to your brain and whole body, boosting the immune system.

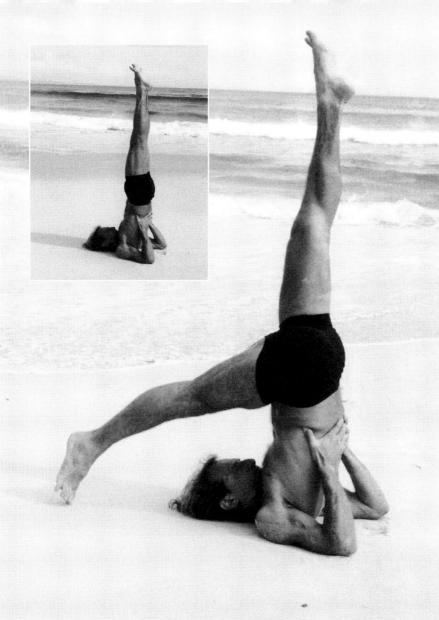

EKA PADA
SARVANGASANA

147

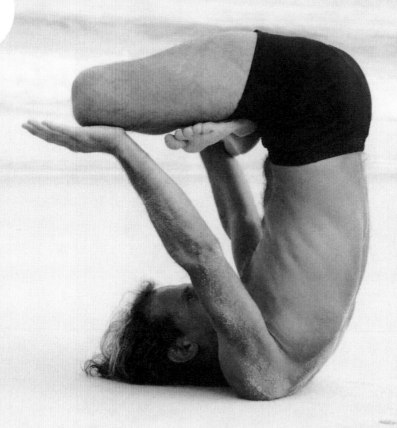

URDHVA PADMASANA
URDHVA – ELEVATED; *PADMA* – LOTUS

This inverted lotus position symbolizes your individual soul's
journey to unite with the universal soul.

POSITIONING: From *Salamba Sarvangasana* (inset photo page 147) bend your
right leg and bring your right foot down to rest on top of your left thigh. Flick your
left foot to cross over the right and rest on top of your right upper thigh. Come into
full *Padmasana*, maintaining the lift in your shoulders and chest. Keep the pressure
on your head light so that there is no strain on the neck. Drop your legs and bring
your hands around to support your knees with your palms. Keep your arms straight
and your chin tucked in. Keep your thighs parallel to the floor, your back lifted and
your shoulders rounded.

FOCUS: Centering your body weight evenly on your shoulders.

GAZE: At the tip of your nose.

BREATHING: Cultivate the sound of your breath moving from the back of your
throat.

HOLD: 25 long, full breaths.

BENEFITS: Increases circulation to your glands; calms your
nervous system; helps relieve headaches; rests your heart and lungs;
increases the blood flow to your brain and whole body, boosting the
immune system; stretches your legs, hips and knees.

PARSVA SARVANGASANA
PARSVA – SIDEWAYS; *SARVANGA* – WHOLE BODY

This twisting inversion requires focused direction of your body weight to maintain balance and equilibrium.

POSITIONING: From *Salamba Sarvangasana* (inset photo page 147), slide your palms down your back and drop your buttocks and hips into your outstretched palms. Use your hands to support your hips and hold your legs so the feet are at eye level. Rest your elbows and upper arms firmly on the floor and allow your hips and buttocks to relax into your hands. This is *Viparita Karani* (as shown in inset photo). Release your left hand to the floor and turn your right hand outward to the right. Keep your buttocks and hips dropping into your right palm and your head in the same position. Rotate the front of your torso and your legs to the right and keep sinking your sacrum and hips into your right hand. Lengthen your legs dynamically out to the right and begin to lower them toward the floor. Point out through your toes, your legs strongly activated. Keep your chin tucked in and use your left arm on the floor for support and balance as you hold.

FOCUS: Activating your legs and keeping them lowered over your right hand; keeping your head straight.

GAZE: At the tip of your nose.

BREATHING: Long, slow, even breaths through your nose.

HOLD: 10 breaths, then release back to center and twist to the left.

BENEFITS: Stretches your abdominal area and spine; stimulates digestion; strengthens your legs; rests your head and heart.

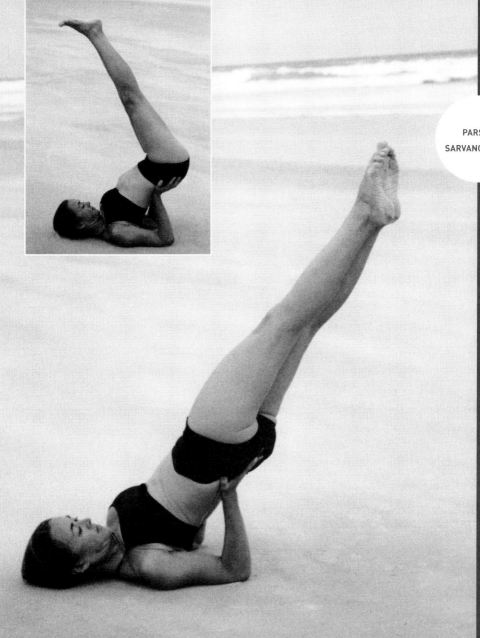

PARSVA
SARVANGASANA

151

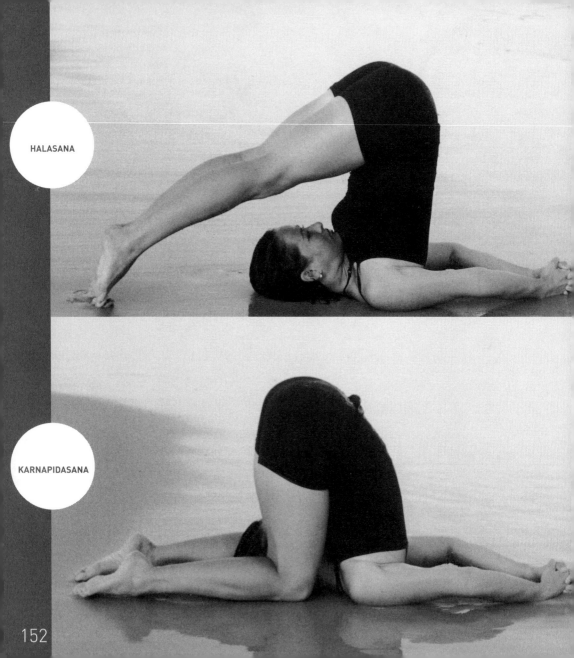

HALASANA

KARNAPIDASANA

152

HALASANA
HALA – PLOUGH

Shut out sounds and distractions and retreat deeply within.

POSITIONING: From *Salamba Sarvangasana* (inset photo page 147), lower your extended legs, resting your toes on the floor. Interlock your fingers behind your back, extending your arms out, and roll onto the top of your shoulders. Lift up through your back, drawing in your lower back and keeping awareness through your legs. Keep your chin tucked in; relax the facial muscles.

FOCUS: Keeping your back and the skin on your back lifting; relaxing your neck and face.

GAZE: At the tip of your nose.

BREATHING: Softly and slowly.

HOLD: 20 breaths or more.

BENEFITS: Quiets your mind; calms your nervous system; nourishes your hormonal system; soothes your head and heart.

KARNAPIDASANA
KARNA – EAR; *PIDA* – PRESSURE

There is nowhere to go, nothing to do. Be here; just you and your breath.

POSITIONING: From *Halasana* (see above), drop your knees beside your ears. Rest your lower legs to the floor and press them into your ears to close out sounds. Allow the weight of your buttocks to drop your knees deeper to the floor. Keep the arms extended back behind you with the palms down or fingers interlocked.

FOCUS: Closing your ears to outer sound; keeping the chin tucked in.

GAZE: Close your eyes to journey deeper inward.

BREATHING: Listen to the soft sound of your breath.

HOLD: 20 breaths or longer.

BENEFITS: Quiets the mind; calms the nervous system; relaxes the heart and organs.

PARTNER POSES

The challenge of Extreme Yoga provides a perfect opportunity to develop our practice in new ways. As we journey more deeply into our personal yoga asana practice, we often reach points when we wish to share our understanding of yoga with others. During these times we can benefit from opening our personal practice up to become a shared one. By joining with another in practice we create a space not only to pass on our own understanding and awareness of yoga, but also to learn from someone else's experience. We discover a new process of development through yoking our physical limitations and strengths with another, adding depth to our tangible experience of yoga. Partner yoga provides new challenges to our practice as we move beyond our usual boundaries to find balance, harmony and lightness in the postures, developing self-awareness and awareness of others. During this process, we develop and refine our communication skills and discover a sense of how we are connected. We experience yoga in its true essence: that of unity. We also discover within us innate intelligence, healing powers and teaching skills as we're forced to reach out to support and assist others in the practice. When working in pairs, allow time for tuning into each other's breath (a back to back sitting position is good), then progress to your chosen postures. Try to maintain synchronized breathing and only practice what feels right for both of you. Ideally you and your partner will have similar heights and levels of flexibility and strength; however, this is not essential. Practice with openness, creativity and care and enjoy the journey beyond self-practice.

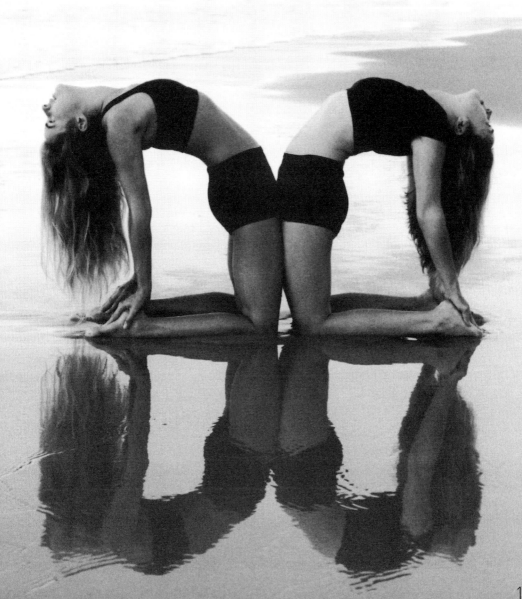

SEATED ON AIR

Rest in calm as you sit in mid-air, relying on each other's strength and support for balance.

POSITIONING: This pose is normally practiced up against a wall, but in this case you become a wall of support for your partner and they for you. Stand with your feet hip-width apart and your back pressing against your partner's. As you exhale, bend your knees and release down, walking your feet out until your lower legs form a right angle with your upper legs, hips in line with your knees, and knees in line with your ankles. Tuck your tailbone under and press firmly into each other's back for support. Link arms for support, rest your hands on your knees, or try raising your arms above your head and joining hands.

FOCUS: Strengthen the legs and stay seated.

GAZE: Softly forward at eye level.

BREATHING: Inhale and exhale softly and evenly through the nose while maintaining the pose.

HOLD: 10 breaths or as long as is comfortable. To release, walk your feet in as you slide up to standing.

BENEFITS: Strengthens the muscles of the legs and knee joints; tones the back and abdominal muscles; develops focus and coordination.

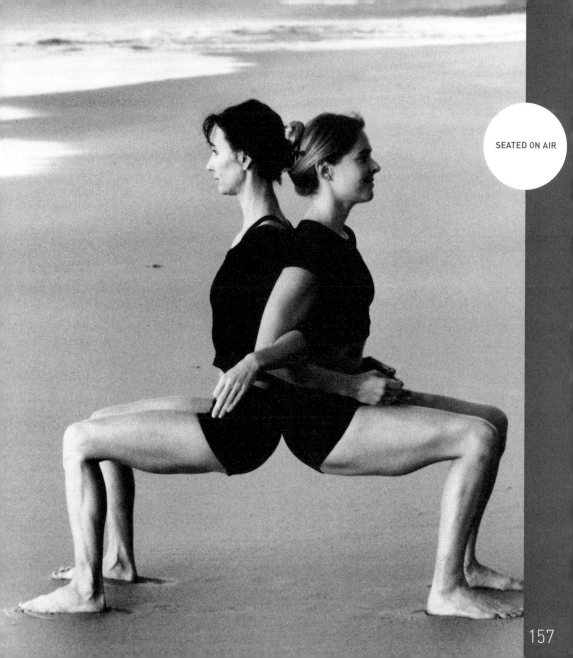

NAVASANA BALANCE
NAVA - BOAT

Floating in calm, mirroring each other's strength, focus and balance.

POSITIONING: Sit opposite your partner, legs outstretched. Raise your legs and bring your feet together. Hold each other's hands around the outside of your legs. On the inhalation breath, pull back away from each other and straighten your legs until they are fully extended. If you cannot come up this way, raise one leg at a time, joining your feet at the top. Draw your lower back in, creating a strong, straight back, and activate your abdominal muscles to support you in the pose. Maintain a central point of balance as you pull away from each other.

FOCUS: Concave your lower back.

GAZE: Softly at your partner.

BREATHING: Soft, even, synchronized breathing.

HOLD: 5–10 deep, full breaths, then release, rest and repeat twice.

BENEFITS: Tones the spinal nerves; strengthens the abdominal muscles, spine, legs and arms; activates the abdominal organs and stimulates digestion; promotes a sense of balance, coordination and focus.

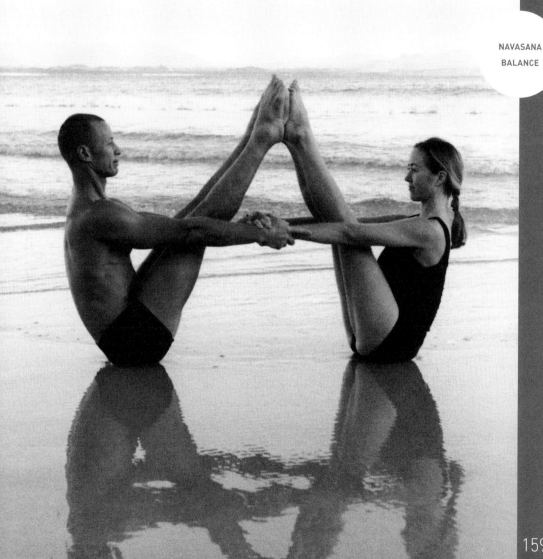

NAVASANA OPENING
NAVA - BOAT

Extending up and outward, create equilibrium with grace.

POSITIONING: Sit opposite your partner, your legs outstretched. Raise your feet up to meet each other's, bringing your hands together between your legs. Keeping a firm grip with your hands, pull away from each other, straightening your legs and locking your feet against each other. Draw your lower back in and up, and keep your back straight.

FOCUS: Keep your lower back pulled in, your spine lifting and your legs locked.

GAZE: Softly at your partner.

BREATHING: Inhale and exhale softly and evenly.

HOLD: 5-10 deep, full breaths, then release, rest and repeat twice.

BENEFITS: Strengthens the abdominal muscles and activates the abdominal organs; stimulates digestion; tones the spinal nerves and strengthens the spinal muscles; strengthens the legs and arms; promotes a sense of balance, coordination and focus.

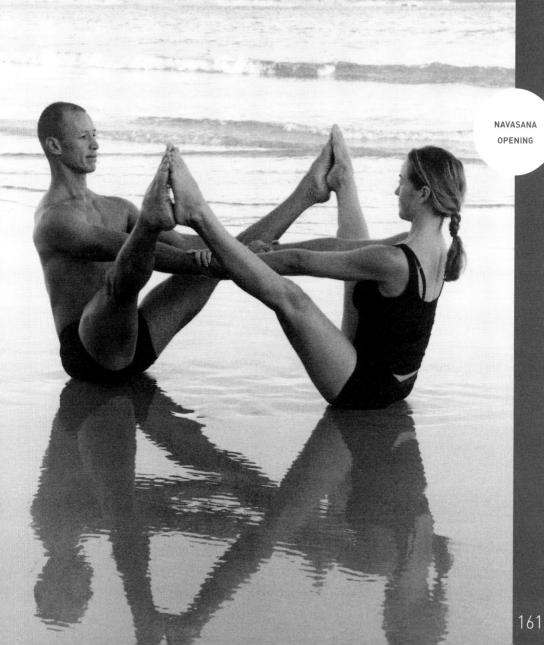

PADMASANA YOKING
PADMA—LOTUS

Two halves create a whole in this beautifully bound embrace.

POSITIONING: Sit facing your partner in full lotus position (see *Padmasana*, pages 30–31). Draw your knees in close together and your feet in close to your groin, flexing your feet. Put your arms behind you on the floor, lean back into them and raise your knees off the floor. Wriggle in close to your partner so that your buttocks and legs press together. One at a time, wrap your arms around your partner's shoulders and draw into each other to form an egg shape with your two bodies.

FOCUS: Lift out of your lower back, keeping your knees close together.

GAZE: Softly at your partner.

BREATHING: Take slow, even breaths through your nose.

HOLD: 5–10 breaths, or as long as is comfortable, then release and cross the legs the opposite way to repeat, or move straight into the *Flowering Padmasana* on the next page.

BENEFITS: Stretches the knee joints; opens the hips; stimulates blood flow to the pelvic region.

NOTE: Only attempt this posture if you're able to sit in *Padmasana* comfortably.

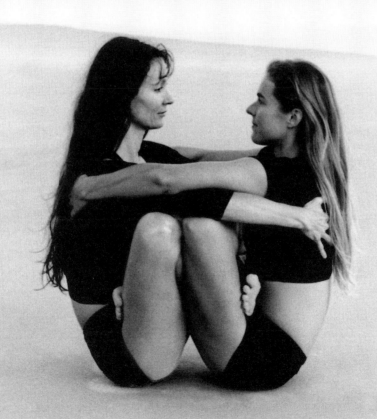

FLOWERING PADMASANA
PADMA—LOTUS

Opening out to life, a blooming flower sprouting from a stable base.

POSITIONING: Position into *Padmasana Yoking*, on the previous page, this time with the arms extended and holding each other's upper arms. Take a deep inhalation together, and on the exhalation drop your head back, pulling away from each other. You may need to release your arms a little. Open your chest, heart and lungs and stretch your throat.

FOCUS: Lift out of your lower back, keeping your knees close together.

GAZE: Focus on your third eye (the point between your eyebrows).

BREATHING: Take deep, full breaths.

HOLD: 5–10 breaths, or as long as is comfortable, then exhale to release. Cross your legs the other way and repeat.

BENEFITS: Stretches the knee joints; opens the hips; stimulates blood flow to the pelvic region; opens the chest and stretches the throat.

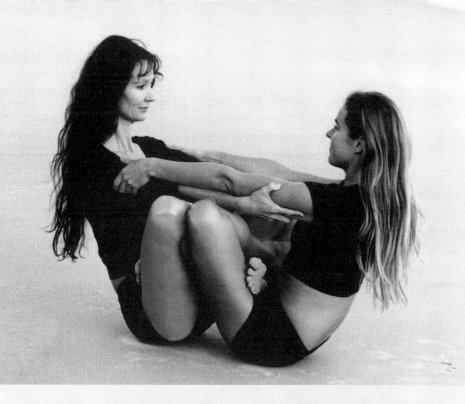

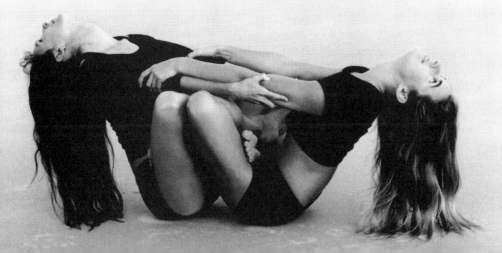

165

KAPOTASANA DOUBLES
KAPOTA—PIGEON

The whole front of the body rounds outward in this intense backward arch.

POSITIONING: One person comes into the full posture, which is the more intense back arch, while the second person rests on the top in the easy variation. Kneel back to back with your partner, your feet and knees hip-width apart and the tips of your toes touching your partner's. First person: inhale to lift out of your lower back and exhale to drop your head back and release your arms over your head to rest your hands on your partner's feet or legs (whichever you can reach). Second person: inhale and then exhale to drop back and rest your hands on your partner's torso (wherever is comfortable).

FOCUS: Keep your hips above your knees, lift and puff your chest outward.

GAZE: Focus on your third eye (the spot between your eyebrows).

BREATHING: Inhale to lift out of your lower back; exhale to soften and arch further back.

HOLD: 5–10 breaths, or for as long as is comfortable, then release up and rest in a forward stretch to counter-pose the backbend before changing positions.

BENEFITS: Tones the spinal muscles and spinal cord; promotes a healthy, supple back; opens the chest, heart and lungs; stimulates blood flow to the pelvic region.

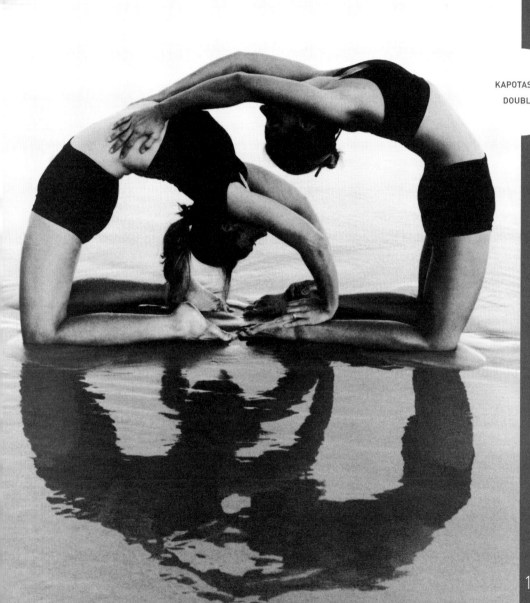

UPSIDE DOWN AND DYNAMIC

Experiment with varying degrees of inversion and develop confidence as you play with upside-down postures.

POSITIONING: One partner goes into the Adho Mukha Svanasana position: kneel on the floor and extend forward. Stretch your arms and spread your fingers wide, your middle finger pointing forward. Step your right foot back, then your left. Straighten your legs, your feet hip-width apart. Inhale and raise your buttocks and hips high; extend your spine upward. Lower the crown of your head downward.

As for the second partner, you will be balancing on your partner's sacrum to apply a gentle lift. To come into the pose, sit in front of your partner in a squatting position until they are in position. Place your hands flat on the floor and when your partner is ready, raise one leg at a time and rest the balls of your feet on their sacral area. Lock your legs and roll your shoulders out, then lock your elbows and lift upward to create a 90° angle with your torso and legs. Lightly move your feet upward to lengthen your partner's spine.

FOCUS: Maintain balance and keep your legs and arms locked.

GAZE: Toward your feet.

BREATHING: Inhale and exhale evenly for balance and steadiness in the postures.

HOLD: 10 breaths, or for as long as is comfortable for both partners. Then swap positions.

BENEFITS: Elongates the spine; stretches the hamstring muscles; tones the legs and arms; stimulates the flow of oxygenated blood to the brain; restorative effect on the heart.

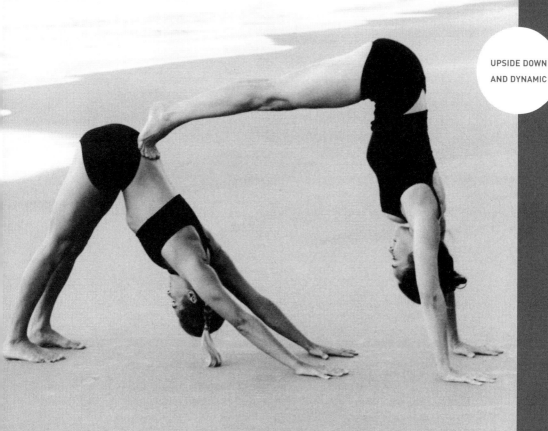

169

8

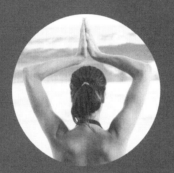

RELAXATION POSTURES

ONE OF THE MOST BEAUTIFUL COMPENSATIONS OF LIFE IS THAT

NO MAN CAN TRULY HELP ANOTHER BEFORE FIRST HELPING THE SELF.

RALPH WALDO EMERSON

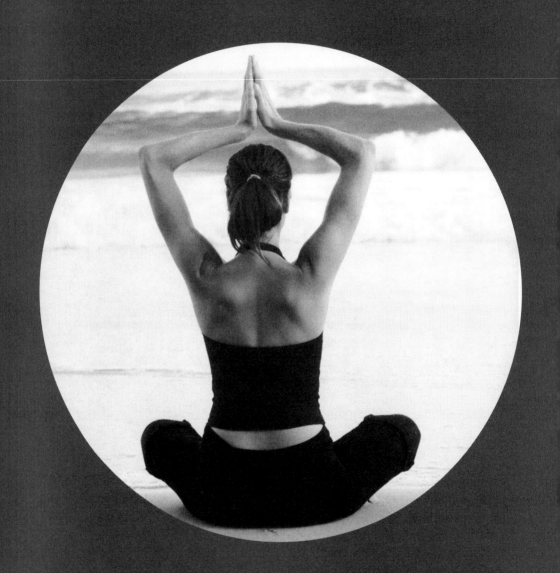

JOURNEY TO RELAXATION

Relaxation yoga postures teach you to relax at will. Whenever you are stressed, exhausted and overworked, you can lie or sit in a relaxation posture with breath focus and gently come back to a space of inner calm. Cultivating the art of relaxation keeps your body's systems healthy and tension-free, helping to prevent the onset of stress-related illnesses and fatigue.

Finding your self in relaxation allows you to rest the soft tissues of your whole body, release tension in your organs, quiet your mind's internal chatter and turn your awareness inward. It is in this quiet internal space that you find a place of oneness. With an open heart and peaceful mind, and as the quiet grows within, you can get in touch with your true self and unearth the passions in your life. There to discover is an endless deep haven of warmth and self-love, which radiates out to others and the world.

Not a lot of physical effort is required for relaxation postures – in fact, the less effort you make, the better. What is required, and can be challenging, is the ability to relax mentally. When the mental effort is reduced and your body is completely tension-free, you experience a delicious sensation of softness throughout your entire being.

To enhance this journey to relaxation, practice away from any distractions. Take the phone off the hook, shut the door to your room, or settle in a shaded space in the garden or by the sea, allowing nature's songs to take you deeper into this restful state.

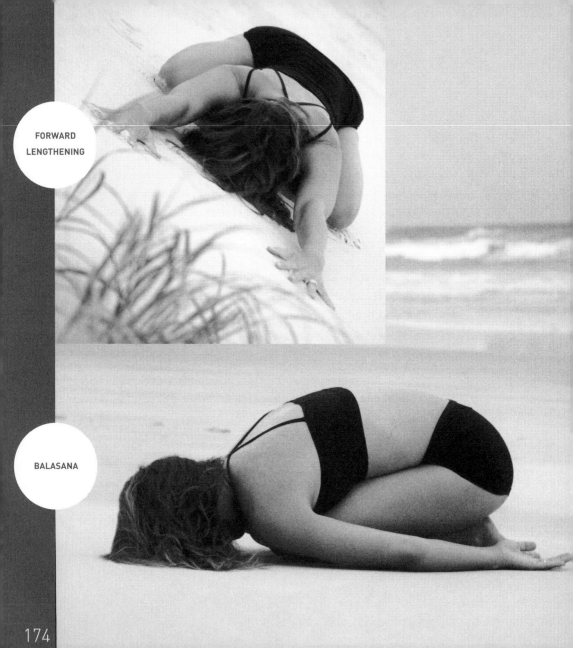

FORWARD
LENGTHENING

BALASANA

174

FORWARD LENGTHENING

Turn inward and allow your nervous system a calm and easy
journey to relaxation.

POSITIONING: Sit with your big toes together, knees wide, with your
buttocks resting on the soles of your feet. Cup your fingers on the floor in
front of your legs. Inhale to lengthen from the front of the torso; exhale to
release forward, stretching your arms out and resting your forehead on the floor.
Sink into relaxation.

FOCUS: Relaxing fully; keeping your buttocks on your heels.

GAZE: Close your eyes for deep relaxation.

BREATHING: Soft breathing for deep relaxation.

VARIATION: Use a bolster or cushion to support your head if needed.

BENEFITS: Lengthens the spine; increases circulation to your organs; relaxes the body
and mind.

BALASANA
BALA – CHILD

Curled up like a small child, we turn our back to the world to find peace within.

POSITIONING: Kneel on the ground; knees and feet together, buttocks resting on the
heels; forehead on the ground in front of the knees, and arms alongside the hips with the
palms face up. Allow the shoulders to drop and close your eyes. Consciously relax the
whole body.

FOCUS: On soft breathing and letting go completely – there is nowhere to go, nothing
to do.

GAZE: Eyelids closed.

BREATHING: Feel your belly softly rising and expanding with the in and out
breaths.

HOLD: As long as desired to quiet the mind and find peace within.

VARIATION: Rest the forehead onto a blanket for comfort; spread the
knees wide if needed.

BENEFITS: Calms your mind; relaxes your head; soothes the
nervous system; "cools" the body's other systems.

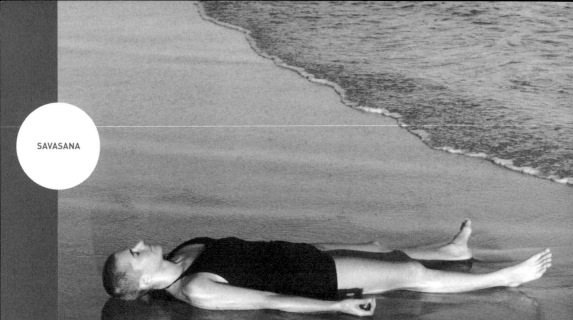

SAVASANA
SAVA – A CORPSE OR LIFELESS BODY

Relax your whole body into the floor and become heavy like a dead weight, a lifeless body.

POSITIONING: Lie flat on the floor with your whole body relaxed; feet falling away from each other; arms out to the side with your palms facing upward. Tuck your chin in, lengthening the back of your neck. Close your eyes and have your lips softly touching to relax your jaw and throat. Relax the muscles around your eyes, eyeballs, forehead and neck. Release any tension in your body completely. Now bring your awareness to the air moving in and out of your nostrils, and the gentle rise and fall of your chest. Without controlling your breath, just observe the air flow. This point of focus helps to let go of thinking and empty your mind.

FOCUS: Consciously relaxing your whole body and following the air flow.

Hold: For 10–20 minutes after a yoga *asana* practice, or whenever you feel the need to relax.

BENEFITS: Relaxes the mind, nervous system – the whole body. Restores energy levels, helps overcome fatigue, insomnia and stress.

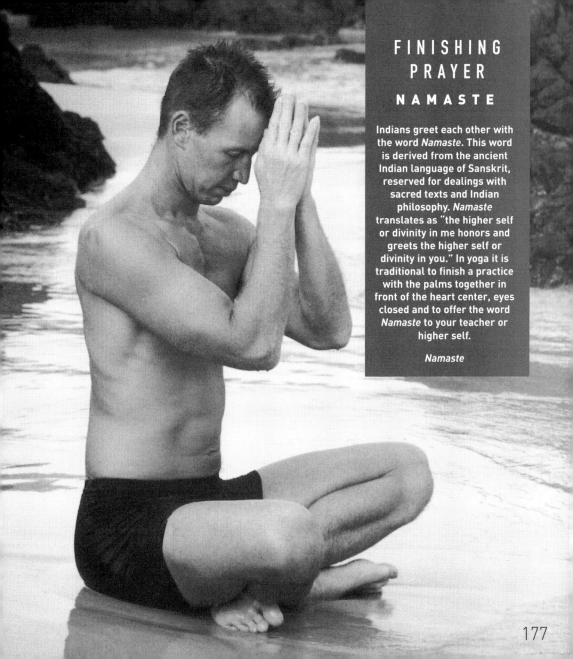

FINISHING PRAYER
NAMASTE

Indians greet each other with the word *Namaste*. This word is derived from the ancient Indian language of Sanskrit, reserved for dealings with sacred texts and Indian philosophy. *Namaste* translates as "the higher self or divinity in me honors and greets the higher self or divinity in you." In yoga it is traditional to finish a practice with the palms together in front of the heart center, eyes closed and to offer the word *Namaste* to your teacher or higher self.

Namaste

177

ACKNOWLEDGMENTS

Most notable thanks go to the unique bird life and stunning sunsets and sunrises that graced the beaches each day, making these images stunning works of art. Dhyan, once again many thanks for the beautiful images of us all in yoga. Your dedication to the project is very inspiring. The yoga models were lovely to work with, easily capturing the essence of the postures and expressing beautifully the art of yoga — thank you! I wrote the majority of this book while teaching a yoga training course in Bali. It was during this time that the bomb went off in Kuta. It was awe-inspiring to be a part of such an incredible show of strength and unity amongst the volunteers who rushed together to be of total service and help save lives and deal with the disaster. The local Indonesian people, expatriates and many tourists worked together tirelessly for days and weeks. During this tragedy I humbly learned what inner strength and endurance are. The focus of this book is developing and cultivating inner strength, and Bali taught me that inner strength is not simply strength, willpower and dynamism, but is also soft, quiet and yielding. The spirit of the Balinese people expressed this most beautifully when, in the face of the bombing, they asked the world not to focus on the death, the terrorism or even retribution but rather to use the opportunity to move more deeply into world peace and unity.

I wish to thank all of the team at HarperCollins, especially Helen Littleton, Associate Publisher, my editor Ali Orman, Lucy Tumanow-West for the copy edit, Jan Hutchinson for proofing, Catherine Day for her help, Justine O'Donnell and Gayna Murphy for the design.

And last but not least *Namaste* to the many inspirational and passionate yoga teachers I have learned, and continue to learn and grow, from.

ABOUT THE AUTHOR

Jessie Chapman is an experienced yoga teacher and Australia's bestselling yoga author. Her books include *Yoga in Focus*, *Yoga Therapies*, *Partner Yoga* and now *Extreme Yoga*. Jessie teaches workshops, trainings and programs internationally and is director of the renowned Radiance Retreats (www.radianceretreats.com), three- to seven-day residential yoga wellness retreats held in Bali and Australia. Since discovering yoga in 1991, she continues to explore and draw inspiration from its varied methods and disciplines, seeing yoga as an ever-evolving and transformational journey of self-discovery and awareness. Her teaching focuses on fullness of breath, fluid unstrained movement, building inner strength, suppleness, balance, natural alignment, vitality, presence and stillness. Email: jessie@intoyoga.com

ABOUT THE PHOTOGRAPHER

Dhyan Dennis has done the photography for all four of Jessie's yoga books. He enjoys the creative exploration involved in capturing the essence and beauty of the postures and loves to be outdoors, especially by the sea. He is a passionate surfer and lives mainly in Byron Bay and Bali. Dhyan has been taking photographs for over 20 years, his favorite subjects being nature and especially flowers, dolphins and birds, as well as exotic faces and places from his many years of travel through Asia and the rest of the world. Dhyan is also an artistic builder and designs beautiful Indonesian-inspired houses. Email: dhyandennis@yahoo.com

ABOUT THE YOGA MODELS

 Pete Watkins is a Capoeira instructor and personal fitness trainer. He is based in Byron Bay.

 Louisa Sear is a yoga teacher and director of Yoga Arts. She teaches classes and retreats in Byron Bay, Australia and around the world. Yoga Arts offers world-renowned 9 months and 2 months yoga teacher training courses in Byron Bay and Bali.

 Lucy Roberts is a yoga teacher based near Byron Bay where she runs Funky Forest Fasts — three-day yoga and fasting nature retreats.

 Pamela Luther teaches yoga in Australia, Hawaii and the Americas. Her passion for travel, snow and surf sees her globetrotting a lot and enables her to study with some of the world's most respected teachers. She also travels to India for cultural and spiritual yoga insights.

 Simon Borg-Olivier is a yoga teacher, physiotherapist and co-director of the Yoga Synergy schools in Sydney. Simon conducts Applied Anatomy for Yoga courses and offers a Synergy yoga teacher training course in Sydney.

Alicia Amore is a professional dancer and has been studying and practicing body movement and yoga for many years. She is passionate about the healing arts and personal development as well as acting and creative dance. She is based in Sydney.

Jessie Chapman is creator of this book and teaches yoga mainly in Australia and different parts of Asia including Byron Bay, her home base. She's operator of Radiance Yoga Wellness Retreats, teaches Yoga Teacher Training Courses and specializes in designing yoga programs.

Pelican is a free spirit currently based on the north coast of NSW. She is passionate about flying and catching fish. This is her first yoga assignment and she looks forward to continued projects on or offshore.

Seagulls are our bird friends who have shown great discipline in turning up at nearly all early-morning photo shoots. They are very advanced yoga practitioners, sometimes spending all day balancing on one leg while maintaining a relaxed composure. This is their fourth yoga book.

INDEX

A

Adho Mukha Svanasana, 14–15
Adho Mukha Vrksasana, 136–137
Adho Mukha Vrksasana variation, 136–137
Ahimsa, 3
Akarna Dhanurasana, 86–87
Aparigraha, 4
arched Supta Virasana, 104–105
Ardha Padmasana, 28–29
arm-balancing postures, 62–83
  Astavakrasana, 70–71
  Bhujapidasana, 66–67
  Dandasana lift, 64–65
  Dwi Pada Sirsasana balance, 82–83
  Eka Hasta Bhujasana, 72–73
  Eka Pada Sirsasana balance, 80–81
  Mayurasana, 76–77
  Tittibhasana – Bakasana sequence, 68–69
  Urdhva Kukkutasana, 78–79
  Vasisthasana II, 74–75
Asana 2, 3, 5, 9–10
Astavakrasana, 70–71
Asteya, 3
"AUM," 32, 45, 50
awareness, developing, 10

B

backward-bending postures,110–123
  Eka Pada Rajakapotasana, 118–119
  Eka Pada Setu Bandha, 112–113
  Kapotasana, 122–123
  Natarajasana, 120–121
  Urdhva Dhanurasana I, 114–115
  Urdhva Dhanurasana II, 116–117
Bakasana sequence, Tittibhasana, 68–69
Balasana, 174–175
Bhujapidasana, 66–67

Brahmacharya, 4
Breathing, 2, 5, 9, 10, 12, 13, 17, 19–22, 35

C

cat curls, 36–37
Caturanga Dandasana, 14–15
comfort, 16
concentration, 2, 6, 9, 24, 32
core strengthening sequence, 40–41

D

Dandasana lift, 64–65
deep full breathing, cultivating, 19–22
dharana, 2, 3, 6, 24, 32
dhyana, 2, 3, 6, 24, 32
Dwi Pada Sirsasana, 108–109
Dwi Pada Sirsasana balance, 82–83

E

Eka Hasta Bhujasana, 72–73
Eka Pada Rajakapotasana, 118–119
Eka Pada Sarvangasana, 146–147
Eka Pada Setu Bandha, 112–113
Eka Pada Sirsasana, 98–99
Eka Pada Sirsasana balance, 80–81

F

finishing prayer, see Namaste
flowering Padmasana, 164–165
forward lengthening, 124, 174–175
forward-bending postures, 124–133
  Kurmasana, 128–129
  Malasana, 130–131
  Skandasana, 132–133
  Upavistha Konasana, 126–127

G

Garbha Pindasana, 92–93
getting started, 13
greeting, 35

H

Halasana, 152–153
Hanumanasana, 94–95

I

Indian philosophy, 2, 3, 177
inner strength, vi–vii, 5, 8, 10, 62, 100, 135
insight into yoga, 1–6
inverted postures, 134–153
  Adho Mukha Vrksasana + variation, 136–137
  Eka Pada Sarvangasana, 146–147
  Halasana, 152–153
  Kona Sirsasana, 142–143
  Padma Pinca Mayurasana, 138–139
  Parsva Sarvangasana, 150–151
  Salamba Sirsasana II sequence, 144–145
  Urdhva Padmasana, 148–149
  Vrschikasana, 140–141
Isvara Pranidhana, 5

J

Jnana Mudra, 25

K

Kapotasana, 122–123
Kapotasana doubles, 166–167
Kona Sirsasana, 142–143
Krounchasana, 90–91
Kurmasana, 128–129

L

life force, 5, 20
lightness, 16
lying-down postures, 100–109
  arched Supta Virasana, 104–105
  Dwi Pada Sirsasana, 108–109
  Matsyasana, 106–107
  Supta Virasana, 102–103

M

Malasana, 130–131
Marjariasana, 36–37
Masta Tadasana, 14–15
Matsyasana, 106–107
Mayurasana, 76–77
meditation, 2, 6, 9, 24, 32
menstruating, 18, 100, 110, 135

N

Namaste, 177
Natarajasana, 120–121
Navasana balance, 158–159
Navasana opening, 160–161
nervous system, 10, 100, 110
niyamas, 2, 3, 4–5

O

"OM," see "AUM"

P

Padma Pinca Mayurasana, 138–139
Padmasana, 30–31
Padmasana yoking, 162–163
Parsva Hasta Tadasana, 42–43
Parsvakonasana, 14–15
Parsva Sarvangasana, 150–151
partner poses, 154–169
  flowering *Padmasana*, 164–165
  Kapotasana doubles, 166–167
  Navasana balance, 158–159
  Navasana opening, 160–161
  Padmasana yoking, 162–163
  seated on air, 156–157
  upside down and dynamic, 168–169
Pinca Mayurasana, 138–139
postures, see arm-balancing, backward-bending, forward-bending, inverted, lying-down, sitting
potential, v, 2, 4, 9, 135

practice, 16
prana, 5, 10, 20
Pranayama, 2, 3, 5, 10
Pratyahara, 2, 3, 6, 24, 32
props, 16–17, 62, 84, 110, 125, 135

R

Relaxation Postures, 13, 14, 171–176
  Balasana, 174–175
  forward lengthening, 174–175
  Savasana, 176

S

sacred space, 17
safety, 18
Salamba Sirsasana II sequence, 144–145
Samadhi, 3, 6
Samakonasana, 96–97
Sanskrit, 2
Santosa, 4
Satya, 3
Saucha, 4
Savasana, 14, 176
seated on air, 156–157
Siddhasana, 26–27
sitting in stillness, 23–32
sitting postures, 84–99
  Akarna Dhanurasana, 86–87
  Eka Pada Sirsasana, 98–99
  Garbha Pindasana, 92–93
  Hanumanasana, 94–95
  Krounchasana, 90–91
  Samakonasana, 96–97
  Ubhaya Padangusthasana, 88–89
Skandasana, 132–133
Sukhasana, 26–27
Supta Virasana, 102–103
Surya Namaskar A, 44–49
Surya Namaskar B, 50–60
Svadhyaya, 5

T

Tadasana, 14–15
Tapas, 4
Tittibhasana – Bakasana sequence, 68–69
Trikonasana, 14–15

U

Ubhaya Padangusthasana, 88–89
Upavistha Konasana, 126–127
upside down and dynamic, 168–169
Urdhva Dhanurasana I, 114–115
Urdhva Dhanurasana II, 116–117
Urdhva Kukkutasana, 78–79
Urdhva Mukha Svanasana, 14–15
Urdhva Padmasana, 148–149
Uttanasana, 14–15

V

Vasisthasana II, 74–75
Vinyasa, 12–15, 84
Virasana, 28–29
Vrschikasana, 140–141
Vyaghrasana, 38–39

W

warm-up sequences, 33–60
  core strengthening sequence, 40–41
  Marjariasana, 36–37
  Parsva Hasta Tadasana, 42–43
  Surya Namaskar A, 44–49
  Surya Namaskar B, 50–60
  Vyaghrasana, 38–39
winding down, 14

Y

yama, 2, 3–4
yoga, philosophy, 2–6

OTHER ULYSSES PRESS BOOKS

YOGA IN FOCUS: POSTURES, SEQUENCES, AND MEDITATIONS
Jessie Chapman   photographs by Dhyan, $14.95

A beautiful celebration of yoga that's both useful for learning the techniques and inspiring in its artistic approach to presenting the body in yoga positions.

YOGA FOR PARTNERS: OVER 75 POSTURES TO DO TOGETHER
Jessie Chapman   photographs by Dhyan, $14.95

An excellent tool for learning two-person yoga, *Yoga for Partners* features inspiring photos of the paired asanas. It teaches partners how to synchronize their movements and breathing, bringing new lightness and enjoyment to any yoga practice.

YOGA THERAPIES: 45 SEQUENCES TO RELIEVE STRESS, DEPRESSION, REPETITIVE STRAIN, SPORTS INJURIES & MORE
Jessie Chapman   photographs by Dhyan, $14.95

Featuring an inspiring artistic presentation, this book is filled with beautifully photographed sequences that relieve stress, release anger, relax back muscles and reverse repetitive strain injuries.

ASHTANGA YOGA FOR WOMEN: INVIGORATING MIND, BODY, AND SPIRIT WITH POWER YOGA
Sally Griffyn, $17.95

Presents the exciting and empowering practice of power yoga in a balanced fashion that addresses the specific needs of female practitioners.

To order these books call 800-377-2542 or 510-601-8301, fax 510-601-8307, e-mail ulysses@ulyssespress.com, or write to Ulysses Press, P.O. Box 3440, Berkeley, CA 94703. All retail orders are shipped free of charge. California residents must include sales tax. Allow two to three weeks for delivery.